John Forsyth Meigs

# A History of the first Quarter of the second Century of the Pennsylvania Hospital

John Forsyth Meigs

**A History of the first Quarter of the second Century of the Pennsylvania Hospital**

ISBN/EAN: 9783337161354

Printed in Europe, USA, Canada, Australia, Japan

Cover: Foto ©ninafisch / pixelio.de

More available books at **www.hansebooks.com**

# A HISTORY

OF THE

# FIRST QUARTER OF THE SECOND CENTURY

OF THE

# PENNSYLVANIA HOSPITAL.

READ BEFORE THE BOARD OF MANAGERS AT THEIR STATED
MEETING HELD 9TH MO. 25TH, 1876.

BY

J. FORSYTH MEIGS, M.D.

Published by the Board of Managers.

PHILADELPHIA:
COLLINS, PRINTER, 705 JAYNE STREET.
1877.

# PREFACE.

In the year 1851, Dr. George B. Wood prepared, at the request of the Managers of the Pennsylvania Hospital, a history of the first hundred years of the Institution.

At the close of the year 1875, the Managers, in view of the approaching celebration in the year 1876, in this city, of the hundredth year of the nation, deemed it wise to have the history of the Hospital continued to that period. The following sketch of the first quarter of the second century of the Institution (1851–1876) is the fruit of this action of the Managers.

In preparing this history, the writer has endeavored to demonstrate to the reader the strict integrity and the close economy with which the affairs of the Institution have been administered. By doing this he hoped to show that to this Hospital, the charitable might safely entrust their gifts, in the sure confidence that their offering would not be lost nor misapplied.

J. FORSYTH MEIGS.

# ADDRESS.

At a stated meeting of the Board of Managers of the Pennsylvania Hospital, held 27th December, 1875, the following preamble and resolutions were adopted:—

*Whereas*, It is believed that benefit would result from bringing up the history of the Pennsylvania Hospital as a supplement to the able Centennial Address delivered by Prof. Wood in 1851, to the present time, thereby furnishing our contributors and fellow-citizens with a correct statement of what has been done by our venerable Institution; and—

*Whereas*, We think there is no one more competent to perform the task than our senior attending Physician, Dr. J. Forsyth Meigs: therefore,

*Resolved*, That he be respectfully invited to undertake the work, in order that we may be kept in remembrance by the very large number of our friends, as well as to make ourselves known to those who are strangers to our just claims upon all who can sympathize with the afflicted.

*Resolved*, That a Committee be appointed to aid Dr. Meigs in obtaining all the information he may require, to furnish a correct list of our officers to

1876, and to superintend the publication. The President named the following members as the Committee, viz.: Alex. Biddle, Joseph B. Townsend, Samuel Welsh, Samuel Mason, T. Wistar Brown.

Signed by the President and Secretary on behalf of the Board.

>WILLIAM BIDDLE, President,
>BENJAMIN H. SHOEMAKER, Secretary.

On receiving notice of the action of the Board of Managers, I gladly undertook the task, having been connected with the Institution for a number of years, first as resident physician, and then as one of the attending physicians, and having always felt towards it a great tenderness and interest.

My predecessor, in writing the history of this noble charity, concluded with the year 1851, the end of the first century of its existence. Those who wish to see from how small a germ this now extensive and most useful Institution has grown, should consult Prof. Wood's interesting address. It carries us back to the days of colonial life, when loyal adherence to the King was one of the moral laws, and when a small town marked the origin of this vast city. It carries us through the war of the Revolution, the separation from the mother country, and the conversion of a colonial Province into a great and independent State, amidst all which changes the Hospital continued its good work, though often under much distress for ways and means.

In 1851 the Hospital, which, up to the year 1841, consisted of but one department, in which the sick and wounded and insane were received and treated in a single building, had been divided for ten years (1841) into two departments, that for the sick and wounded in the city building, and that for the insane at the new establishment in West Philadelphia.

These two departments, I beg the reader clearly to understand, are one and the same Hospital, acting under the one original charter, granted by the Provincial Assembly of the Pennsylvania Province in 1751, managed and governed by the same Board of Managers. The two are but different members of the one body, having the same interests, an equal pride in success, and equal grief in times of distress, each one assisting the other when assistance is needed, and both aiding in the one common object, the relief and cure of the sick, wounded, and insane. These facts I insist upon, because there has been, it is said, a feeling of jealousy in the minds of some, since the separation into two departments, as to the relative importance of the one or the other. And yet this feeling ought not to exist, for in the charter it is written that the Hospital is intended "for the reception and relief of lunaticks, and other distempered and sick now within this Province." The Managers were compelled, therefore, to provide for the care of the insane. The charter, indeed, puts the "lunaticks" first in the order of enumeration. Whether this phraseology of the deed were accidental, as is most probable, or intentional, it is impossible to say. Dr.

Franklin, who had so much to do with the foundation of the Hospital, gives, in his autobiography, a short history of its inception, saying that in 1751, "Dr. Thos. Bond, a particular friend of mine, conceived the idea of establishing a hospital in Philadelphia (a very beneficent design, which has been attributed to me, but was originally his) for the reception and cure of sick persons, whether inhabitants of the Province or strangers." Here we have the germ-idea of the Hospital, and, doubtless, what Drs. Bond and Franklin thought of at the moment was the whole body of sick poor.

At first, all the patients were treated in one building; for who, more than a century ago, understood the true methods of treatment and cure of the insane? But, as time went on and knowledge grew, the managers and the medical staff of the Hospital learned, by degrees, that the treatment of insane persons required other accommodations, other surroundings and influences, than those which could be obtained within the narrow bounds of one square of ground, in the heart of a great city.

But all this will be told hereafter. What I now wish again to impress upon the reader, is the fact that the Hospital is but one, and that my duty will be to trace the history of its two departments from the year 1851, the end of the first century of its existence, to the present year 1876, the first Centennial year of the nation.

In the year 1851, when my history is to begin, ten years after the separation of the two departments, the

Managers were busily engaged in completing some very important changes in the city Hospital, to fit it for what was, in the future, to be its portion of the great work of the Institution, the care of the sick and wounded. Already, the west wing, which, prior to the year 1841, was devoted to the insane patients, had been completely remodelled, so as to make two admirable wards, the lower story devoted to the Women's Surgical, the upper to the Women's Medical wards. The long corridors connecting the centre building with the western wing, are built with alcoves on each side, each alcove containing two beds, and allowing the inmates, by means of a curtain hung across the opening into the corridor, to enjoy a certain amount of privacy, the possession of which is to some of the more sensitive patients a great luxury.

Each of these wards has its own bath-rooms, water-closets, and a ward-kitchen, in which latter can be prepared any special food that may be necessary.

In 1851, the west wing was, as I have said, finished, and the centre building also had been greatly modified. Amongst other changes, the new Library had been built, from what had been previously the Women's Medical Wards. The east wing was being remodelled. The long ward, connecting the centre with the wing fronting on Eighth Street, was taken down, and the two long wards erected, as they now stand. These wards have no alcoves like those of the west wing. The east wing was not taken down, but considerable changes were made in it. This part of the house was devoted to the male patients, the lower stories to surgical, and the upper to medical patients. They are excellent wards, and are heated, ventilated, and provided with bath-rooms, water-closets, and kitchens like the west wing. The repairs to, and other changes, made in the centre building, and the east wing, in 1851 and 1852, cost $59,949.59. The cost of repairing the west wing in 1846–47 was $17,865.28, and that of fitting up the library was $3146.35. The latter expense was paid out of the medical fund.

Another change made in 1851 was the closing of the lying-in ward, at first for the purpose of making room for the other patients during the repairs to the main buildings. The ward was finally closed by a vote of the Board in 1853. It had cost $20,000 more than its whole fund, principal and interest. Moreover, there had been several recurrences of puerperal fever amongst the patients, and it was feared that these visitations had some connection with the surgical wards, and possibly with the post-mortem examinations, which the resident physicians were compelled to make.

Besides the centre and main buildings there is quite a large house in the northeastern portion of the hospital square, which has long been known as the North House. This building has three stories, and has had for many years a ward for syphilitic cases, and another for colored male patients. Within a very few years, as I shall have occasion to tell, one of the lower rooms of this house has been converted into a Recent-Accident ward. This building has its own proper bath-rooms, water-closets, and kitchen. It is even now proposed to pull down this old and not conveniently arranged building, and remodel and enlarge it, or to erect a new one to serve its present purposes, and to be used also for the out-door patient or dispensary department, which has grown into very considerable importance within a few years past. On the northwestern portion of the square is another quite large building, which was originally a stable and cow-house, the upper story of which has been fitted up into wards which, though low, imperfectly lighted, heated, and ventilated, can be, and have been, temporarily used to receive the patients from the other wards, when the latter had to be vacated for the purpose of cleaning, painting, or repairs. The building on Spruce Street, which had been erected to receive West's famous picture of Christ healing the sick, was, when this picture was removed to the Academy of Fine Arts, leased to the College of Physicians. When the College removed to their new building, the picture-house, as it was called, was leased to the Historical Society.

I pass on now to the general history of the city department of the Hospital, that for the sick and wounded, during the last twenty-five years (since 1851). In doing this I shall show that this department has been on the whole growing steadily in usefulness, and in its means for doing good, and I shall show, too, what great difficulties have been met and overcome by the managers—how, during, and since the war, the expenses of the department have constantly outrun the income of the whole vested capital of the institution, and how the managers have been compelled to appeal to the public for the means of paying the annual expenses.

The number of patients received into the wards has been increasing. In the five years from 1851 to 1855 inclusive, the whole number was 8845, of which number 6117 were on the free list, and 1728 were pay patients, making a percentage of 72 free. From 1872 to 1876, inclusive, the whole number received was 9250, of which 7088 were free, and 2163 pay, or 76 percentage of poor.

In the report for the year 1856, the managers call attention to the increasing demands made upon this department, owing to the growth of the population of the city from 20,000, when the Hospital began its career, to 500,000, at that time. They state that, had they the funds to defray the expenses of an increased number of patients, they have ample accommodations for seventy-five additional in the wards. One special cause of the difficulty in which the hospital was now placed for funds, was the singular, and very great, increase in the cost of provisions. The managers state, that within ten years, the outlay for provisions had increased 75 per cent., and yet this was some years before the war began, to which has been generally attributed the rise in the cost of food, which has oppressed us all.

In the same year a Committee on Retrenchment was appointed by the Board. This Committee met several times, and had a synopsis of the statistics of the house, for the previous ten years, prepared by the Steward. From this it appeared "that the number of patients on the poor-list (other than recent accidents) continues to average about seventy daily; there has been no increase of them, while of recent accidents the number has nearly doubled, there being twenty-nine in 1846, since gradually increasing, until now the average is fifty-six. This will partially account for the very greatly increased expenses of the Institution, as such cases are very costly in the appliances used, and the stimulants, medicines, and diet that are required." During this period (1846 to 1856) the number of patients increased from 114 to 166, and the whole number of inmates of the house from 150 to 211. The annual expenditures had been in 1846, $15,909.47; in 1856, they were $36,741.04. The drafts on the Treasurer had increased from $12,200 per annum to $25,000. The Committee concluded that the chief reasons for these largely increased expenditures, were the increased size of the family, the great number of recent accidents, and the high price of provisions and food.

These facts—that the expenses had considerably more than doubled, whilst the number of patients had increased but little over one-third—will explain how difficult a task the Managers had before them. The endowment fund was growing very slowly, but the expenses had more than doubled, and the number of patients increased but little over a third. What were they to do? More money must be raised, and we shall see, as we go on with the history, with what patient courage and perseverance, the Managers continued to press the cause upon the public.

In the Report for 1857, it is again stated that the income of the Hospital is insufficient for its maintenance, and they appeal again forcibly to the public for aid.

We find the same difficulty constantly referred to in the various reports. In that for 1864, regret is again expressed that the means of usefulness of the city department cannot be increased. The doors of the Hospital must remain shut to many for the want of adequate funds. The income of the Hospital, they state, "is reduced, whilst the cost of support of the patients, from the high price of provisions and supplies of all kinds, is much greater than ever before." The cost of fuel alone for the last year had been $11,600 more than for the year prior to that. The Steward of one of the departments, on returning from market, stated that he had just paid $65 for what he formerly obtained for $35.

By this time, things had reached such a climax that the means of the Hospital must be increased, or its expenses diminished. The only possible method of lessening the expenses, would have been to close some of the wards, or to limit to a much lower point than had been the rule, the number of admissions. From the earliest period of the history of the Institution, one invariable practice had obtained in its management, of which the Managers, the Surgical and Medical Staff, the Officers, all its old personal friends, and the whole public of Philadelphia, were proud with a just and noble pride. This was a rule which had never been departed from. It was the law of the house that any recent accident, brought to the Hospital within twenty-four hours of its occurrence, should be received without question. I have never known this law and custom to be infringed. It was known to all classes of Philadelphia citizens. Any laborer, mechanic, engineer, or wayfarer, undergoing a surgical injury within twenty-four hours of Philadelphia, was, until within a very few years, carried by universal acclamation to the Hospital. When I was a mere boy, many times have I seen a wooden settee, bearing some wounded sufferer, lifted upon the shoulders of four men, being carried slowly and carefully through the streets, with its few or many friends attending, and with its train, of course, of inevitable boys. I knew at once what it meant, as did all passers-by. "Ah! some poor fellow has been hurt, and they are taking him to the Hospital."

This being the law and tradition of the Hospital, the Managers had but one course before them: to close the medical wards entirely, or to diminish the number both of medical cases, and of surgical cases, other than recent accidents.

Distant hints began to be given as to the dread necessities which had come upon the old house, and the possible closure of the medical wards was occasionally whispered about.

But the Managers rose to the occasion, as they always had done in the history of this great charity. And I deem myself fortunate in being the man, whose right and duty it is to say, that Philadelphia is justified in the pride she takes in the management of this Institution. And when its citizens shall see, as I am about to show them, how the Managers carried the Hospital over this dreary and dismal time, they may well say, "Well done, good and faithful servants;" and they may, too, justly pride themselves upon their own liberality towards the Hospital on these occasions.

In 1864, at the annual meeting of the contributors in the month of May, the Managers applied for, and received, authority to "appeal to our fellow-citizens in the endeavor to raise an amount sufficient to cover the encroachment on our capital of previous years (which necessity compelled), of some forty thousand dollars, as well as the probable deficiency of the present year, of at least an equal sum, it being supposed there would be an increased expenditure necessary in the cost of living, and the result has shown the correctness of this opinion."

The appeal was made, and, though the applications for money at this time, in consequence of the war, were innumerable, the Managers obtained the sum of $65,055 by contributions. Soon after this, a strong appeal was made by the medical and surgical staff, several thousand copies of which were distributed. Aided by this renewed invitation to the charitable, the Committee raised $34,948.27 additional. Out of this total, $100,003.27, the indebtedness to the capital of $40,000 was refunded, and, after paying the year's (1865) deficiency of $42,000, the surplus of $18,000 was merged in the capital.

But the Hospital was not yet, by any means, through its troubles. In the Report of the Managers for 1866, are some statements, which I shall quote, that its friends may see through what evil times it had to pass during the great rebellion, and with what courage and animation, tempered sometimes with fear and doubt, the Managers fought on through their many difficulties and embarrassments.

This Report (1866) says: "The abnormal condition in which our country has been placed during the past five years, has equally taxed the resources of the Government, and those of our benevolent institutions, depending for their existence and usefulness upon the popular favor and support. Individuals, it is true, have been enriched by the long and exacting war in which the nation has been engaged; and the recently published list of colossal incomes disclosed to the world the names of those who, in this untoward state of things, have been signally benefited by the sectional struggle that has prevailed, but the country at large has become a pecuniary debtor to such a degree that might well appal the stoutest heart in contemplating the possible period of its relief. Besides, there are many individuals around us who have involuntarily changed their relation of creditor to that of debtor, and who mourn unavailingly over a desolation that promises no return to meet their suspended and craving obligations at home. Under these circumstances, it should occasion no surprise that institutions dependent on voluntary aid for their maintenance, should experience the greatest embarrassment in carrying out the purposes of their creation. The abstraction of so many men from the field of production, and the necessary change in the standard of values incident to a protracted war, have augmented prices to such an extent, that the established endowment and current receipts have proved wholly inadequate for the support of our leading charitable institutions."

The Report refers to the well-known fact that there is so often to be seen in the public papers, the short record "sent to the Pennsylvania Hospital," when by some terrible accident, one or two, or even twenty sufferers, have been sent to the surgical wards without announcement, where they have always been received and tended with every care. It refers to the increased costs of the Institution, and says: "But the necessaries of life, and the indispensable appliances in ministering to the afflicted, have advanced more than twofold in price since our civil war began, whilst the number of free or unremunerating patients has largely increased in both the medical and surgical wards. The numbers of the former might be curtailed, and, indeed, the wards might be closed altogether; but this would be a sad alternative, for besides the suffering that would thus be intensified, the character of the Hospital in its connection with our far-famed medical schools would be greatly impaired." Here we see a distinct reference to the possibility of the Managers being forced to close one of the most important wards of the Hospital.

But, fortunately for the poor, for the city, and for

the good fame of the Hospital, the Managers still struggled bravely on.

They, in concert with a Committee of the contributors, issued a strong appeal to the public, stating that "the present current expenses of the Institution require about fifteen thousand dollars per annum more than its income from investments and pay-patients." The number of patients in the Hospital at this time was 171, and of these, 133 were on the free-list. The cost of the Hospital for the fiscal year 1865 was $57,481.32, while the income from investments and from pay-patients had been $42,122.77.

The appeal proposed that subscriptions should be made first for specified sums, to be paid annually for a term of years, towards the deficient income of the Hospital, and, secondly, of sums to be added to the permanent fund, of which the interest or income alone should be used.

In the following year, ending May, 1867, under the appeal just referred to, there were received $20,400 to be added to the capital fund, and $136,556 to be paid by instalments running through periods of three, four, and five years, as contributions to the annual expenses.

With these additions to its means, the department continued its work with comparative ease for a few years. But it was limited as to its usefulness. In the Report of the medical and surgical staff to the Board of Managers, in May, 1869, the staff set forth that "we regret not to be able to report to you from year to year any great increase in the number of patients, as both space and means limit us in that respect. With appropriate buildings and ample pecuniary resources, we could within the square of ground which we occupy, make our Hospital one of many more beds; but, as these are wanting, we must at present be content with the policy of improving and perfecting the accommodations that we already have."

In 1872, the Managers are compelled to express the fear that, as the subscriptions towards the annual expenses, made in 1866-7, were running out, there would again be a heavy deficiency, unless the citizens came forward with additional help. They refer to their difficulties in the following strong language: "We do not hesitate to say that, whilst economy in expenditures has been carefully studied in all that relates to the internal management of the Hospital, we fear that economy has reached the point of parsimony, from an inability to supply the comforts of the suffering."

I can bear witness to the truth of all this, as I was on duty during three months of each year, and I know the economy was what one sees and feels, in the care of a family living on a very straitened income. The Hospital needed many changes and renovations, but as yet the income made it impossible to do more than continue the same average course it had been following for a number of years. The Managers wished to improve the ventilation, renew the household material, provide better maintenance for and attendance upon the sick, and improve the culinary department.

In 1873, the deficiency in the income was still very great, but the Report says that: "As regards the endowment fund—the interest of which is alone applicable to current expenses—it has been pleasing to Providence to place it in the hearts of men voluntarily to increase it by amounts rarely equalled in any year of our existence."

In 1875, this department was still very much embarrassed, though the deficiency was not quite so great as in previous years. The expenses were $65,441.17, an excess over the income from the endowment fund, and the receipts from pay-patients and subscriptions received by the Steward, of over eight thousand dollars ($8,173.69).

In this year many improvements were made at a very large cost. They were shown to be necessary by the light of recent hygienic discoveries.

The Report states that, "in the male department, the windows in the wash-rooms have been enlarged to admit more light and air. New marble basins, with hot and cold water, have been added; new receivers of iron, lined with porcelain, with traps and larger pipes, have been placed in the water-closets, with an increased flow of water for drainage. Bath rooms have been re-arranged, and basins, with marble or slate tops, placed throughout the wards. In the basement a large coil of pipe, heated by steam, has been placed at the lowest part of the main ventilating chimney, to insure the more effectual rarefaction of the air. Two new bath-rooms have been placed in the female department, and all closets, clothes rooms, chambers, kitchens, wards, and halls, after being carefully cleaned, have received several coats of paint; all bath-rooms arranged with larger drainage and increased supply of water, and the floors laid of slate. Stationary wash-tubs have been added in the basement. New iron bedsteads of improved construction have been introduced. The same improvements, with new slate flooring, have been made in the middle building. Refrigerators have been placed in the ward dining-rooms. In the receiving ward, a new bath-tub, washstand, and clothing closet have been supplied. Slate tables have been placed in the dead-house, which has also been partially repainted."

"The out-patient rooms, with the North House, their roofs, and water-supply, have connections for drainage with the sewers. The kitchens have also been renewed, sinks, and hot and cold water introduced. The lodge has been painted, and an iron guard rail been placed to separate the out-patient rooms and their visitors from the interior grounds of the Hospital."

The Board now, too, determined that the time had come when the ventilation of the Hospital for the sick and wounded must be brought to the same perfection as that which had long been attained to in the Insane Department. In 1875, the ventilation continued just as it had been arranged in 1851-2, when these buildings were remodelled and renovated. No changes nor improvements had been made. There had been, of late years, a good many cases of pyæmia in the surgical wards. Some of the principal capital surgical operations had proved fatal; and especially was this true of ovariotomy, and both Managers and staff had become seriously uneasy about the ventilation. Some imperfect attempts had been made to improve the arrangements as they stood, but they were of no real value; and now the Managers "sought the advice of experienced constructors of buildings, where forced ventilation by fans and flues for heated air has proved successful." Indeed, the experience of the Insane Department, as it is ably detailed by the superintendent, was alone enough to convince the Managers, and did largely convince them, that the only thoroughly efficient remedy was to be found in the use of the system of propulsion, by means of a fan.

The use of a fan was finally determined upon, and, in the present year, 1876, the plan has been carried into effect under the supervision of John Sunderland, the former supervisor of the erection of the heating apparatus for the Department for the Insane.

A fan 8 feet in diameter, and 30 inches wide, is placed at the orifice of a large fresh-air duct, which leads to the chamber containing the steam coils for heating, and thence by large smooth flues to all parts of the house. This fan is calculated to supply 30,000 cubic feet of air per minute. Two of my sons calculated the capacity of the large air-duct, and determined the velocity of the current of air passing through it by means of an anemometer. Unfortunately, they did not know that two side ducts had been given off from the main duct, in advance of the point at which they made their observations. But it is of interest to know that, even at this point, the supply of air amounted to 715,800 cubic feet per hour. This, assuming that the population of the house is about two hundred, would give to each person 3575 cubic feet per hour. Dr. Parkes, in his able work on Hygiene, states that for healthy men 3000 cubic feet per hour should be supplied, and for sick men 4000 feet. By the imperfect observation above made, we learn that each patient in the Hospital will receive within 425 cubic feet of the amount of air deemed necessary by one of the highest authorities on this question, and, when we recollect that two ducts had already taken off a considerable amount of the air furnished by the fan, there can be no doubt that the supply of air to the wards will be quite equal to the standard usually deemed necessary.

After this sketch of the general history of the City Hospital, in regard to its financial concerns, and the improvements in its buildings, I proceed to notice various other points of interest in its gradual development. I shall refer particularly to its course as a centre of clinical teaching—to the erection and opening of a new and fine lecture and operating room; to the reception of women as medical students; to the Pathological Museum; to the opening of the Dispensary, or out-door Department, of a Recent Accident Ward, and to the proposition for the endowment of free beds.

And first, as to what the Hospital has been doing in aid of medical education during the last twenty-five years. During the early years of this period, the system of clinical instruction continued to be on the same plan as during the latter part of its first century. Lectures were given twice a week by the physicians and surgeons, as a part of their recognized duties. For the privilege of attending these lectures the fee was ten dollars a year, and the amount received was still applied to the care and increase of the medical library. The classes were large, and the valuable lessons thus imparted, at a merely nominal cost, were open to all men who had matriculated in a respectable medical institution. After a time, it was found that the old lecture room, in the third story of the centre building, had become too small to accommodate the classes with any reasonable comfort, either to listener or teacher. Moreover, the example of the Blockley Hospital, which had provided a large and commodious amphitheatre for clinical teaching, and that of other cities, and still more decidedly the spread of the conviction, from the medical to the lay mind, that the medical art could not be properly taught without extensive clinical opportunities, induced some movement in this Hospital towards better accommodations for the students.

This matter is first distinctly referred to in the Annual Report for 1860, where the Managers express the opinion that, at no distant day, the lecture and operating room must be enlarged. In 1861, a sum of five hundred dollars was given to one of the Managers to be used for the relief of sufferers by the war, should such apply at the Hospital, and, if not thus used, the money was to go towards the commencement of a fund for the enlargement of the lecture room. In 1863, the Managers again say that: "As Philadelphia has hitherto stood pre-eminent for her medical schools, it has been the desire of the successive Boards of Managers of the Hospital to co-operate with their distinguished professors in affording every facility for instruction to the students of medicine and surgery resorting to this city for their education. The extensive and valuable medical library belonging to the Institution is freely accessible to them; but there is a want experienced in the limited accommodations of the lecture and operating room. The present Board trust that, upon the return of peace and of general prosperity, it may be in the power of the Institution to provide more ample conveniences for the increased number of students, who will undoubtedly avail themselves of the extraordinary advantages our city affords for their improvement in the profession they have chosen as their pursuit in life."

In 1867, it is again referred to, but, though the cost would be but about $20,000, the Board did not feel warranted in applying the funds to this purpose, "so long as the income from the capital is insufficient to meet the annual cost of support of the patients."

In 1868, it is stated that a sum of $6990 has been contributed towards this object, and, so convinced are they of its necessity, that the Managers make an "earnest appeal to the contributors to take such action at this meeting, as will enable the Board to proceed at once to the consummation of the purpose which they have long had in view."

Accordingly, authority was given by the contributors for the erection of a new room for clinical and operating purposes.

The site chosen is to the north of the centre building, far enough from this to receive a good light from all points. The building is of brick, octagonal in shape, and has eight double windows in the eastern and western walls, and a large skylight looking to the north. It is connected with the centre building of the Hospital by a corridor, opening into what was previously the main entrance door at the north, and its main floor is on a level with that of the centre. The seats are arranged as in an amphitheatre, rising from the floor of the area where the lecturer stands towards the walls, and they will accommodate about 500 students. On either side of the south end of the building are two small rooms in which the patients can be placed until it is time to take them into the clinic. There is quite a large, well-lighted basement room beneath the northern half of the lecture room, which is devoted to the Pathological Museum of the Hospital, now becoming an important and useful element in the clinical work of the Institution.

This room cost $27,072.10, of which sum $12,742.80 had been raised by specific subscriptions for this purpose.

The Managers, therefore, were obliged to take the deficiency, $14,329.26, from the capital stock. It was formally opened on the ninth of January, 1869, on which occasion I had the honor of making an address to the Managers, the medical and surgical staff, and to the students, to mark the occasion. I chose for my subject the history of clinical teaching, as connected with the Pennsylvania Hospital, and the value of such teaching to the public in general, and to the medical student in particular. I will venture to quote an extract from that discourse: "I believe," I then said, "and I do not hesitate to express my belief, that, in connection with the proper treatment of the sick in a hospital, one of the most beneficent uses of such an institution, is the aid which it can and ought to give in propagating a wise system of medical education. By such a management, two grand results are accomplished. All is done by the Institution that the best and purest charity can effect for the individual sick within its walls, whilst by fitting young men for the difficult and important office of the physician, it radiates from its own narrow centre, to the vast mass of suffering humanity beyond its walls, a knowledge and experience of the best methods of treating wounds and diseases, which is of incalculable value to the public. I know well that there are some benevolent and tender spirits, to whom the idea of making anything like a use of the sick as a means of teaching medicine, savors of something harsh and revolting. But to such as have this very natural and proper fear, I will say that no well-trained and conscientious medical officer ever forgets that his first duty is to the individual sick man intrusted to his charge, and that he is bound in honor and charity to allow no ulterior object to work detriment to him. In all hospitals, there are many cases which can, without danger of injury, be brought before a medical class. Most of the patients, when the matter is properly and kindly represented to them, make no objection to such a procedure. Some rather enjoy it, and gladly lend their mite to the common good. Moreover, it seems but right that those who are fed and housed, and furnished with all the means and advice necessary to their medical treatment by the public, should make this moderate return of assisting, for the public, in the necessary education of competent medical men. Let it not be forgotten, too, that this demonstration is never made to a promiscuous, or rude, or gaping public audience, who might assist at such a spectacle from mere vulgar curiosity. It is made only to those who belong to the same vocation or guild as that to which belong the surgeons and physicians of the house, and but for whom this Hospital could not exist, and who, themselves, but for like opportunities in the past, could not have had that exact knowledge and experience whereby these very patients now profit."

In connection with this matter it ought to be stated that this Hospital has always been in favor of a proper use of its wards for the purposes of medical instruction. It has, from its earliest days, contributed regular clinical lectures by its staff, and it has been frequented by large numbers of students. Indeed, for a long course of years, it was the only Hospital in the city, and the only public ground on which the medical student and the sick man could be properly brought together.

For some years past, however, a change has been taking place as to the clinical opportunities in the city. Other hospitals have been erected which are destined in the future, it seems probable, to diminish the classes of the Pennsylvania Hospital. The Blockley Hospital has, for a number of years, had large classes; and now, that of the two great medical schools, one, the University of Pennsylvania, has already a fine hospital attached to its own foundation, and the other, the Jefferson Medical College, is building one for its own purposes, it is to be expected that our classes must lessen in size. In fact, the number of students in attendance during the session of the schools, has fallen off considerably within the last three years.

Nor do I know that this is to be regretted. It should seem that several classes of moderate size, in which the members of the class can be seated nearer to the patient and the lecturer, must afford better opportunities to the students, than where huge classes are crowded together to observe those delicate phenomena of disease, by the study of which alone can the medical art be properly acquired.

I come now to a new feature in the history of the Hospital. I refer to the introduction of female medical students to the clinical instruction of the institution.

In the autumn of 1869, the Dean of the Faculty of the Female Medical College applied to the Board of Managers for the admission of their students to the regular clinical courses. The Managers gave their permission on the ground that, by the rules of the Hospital then in use, all students of institutions recognized by the State laws, were to be received to the common benefits of the Hospital clinical instruction.

The women came to one of the lectures very soon after this, taking their seats in the amphitheatre in the midst of the regular men's class. There was a scene of considerable disorder both during and after the lecture.

The event caused a good deal of agitation in the medical schools of the city, and amongst the medical students, which extended in a slight degree to the general public. It raised the great questions of women's rights, and of the common education of the sexes. And it showed, too, most clearly, that women were willing, in order to obtain their end, a general medical education and a status in the profession similar to that of men, to listen in mixed classes to descriptions of all diseases, whether medical or surgical, and to observe any class of cases, which might be necessary in the course of their medical education. It was a curious and an impressive lesson, to show how long-established social habits and opinions may be changed by the hard weight of necessity.

It was thought by many that the objection made by the medical students, and by the medical teachers of the old schools of the city, arose wholly from a jealous dislike to the increased competition that might occur in the profession, should women come to participate fully in the exercise of the medical art. I think not. I believe the difficulty lies deeper than this. It is a psychological one, and, strange to say, it appears to exist more decidedly in the male than in the female sex.

In the following clinical session, 1870–71, the whole number of students in attendance was 206, and of these, 32 were women; whilst in the previous year, the number had been 500, of which number 42 were women.

The matter was arranged at the meeting of the contributors, in May, 1871, on the plan of having separate clinics for the two sexes, and, accordingly, the staff agreed to give, in addition to their regular semi-weekly lectures to the male students, one lecture a week to the women students. This plan has been followed since.

I have referred to the diminution in the number of students in the session of 1870–71. The staff and managers were both disturbed at finding the classes falling off so rapidly from the Institution which had long been at the head of clinical teaching in the city. By advice of the staff, the managers determined to make the lectures free "to all students of incorporated institutions recommended by the lecturers," whilst the women students were to be taught, as before mentioned, in a separate class. The consequence of this step was, that the classes increased at the next session to the number of 580, the men counting 520, and the women 60.

As to whether the entire withdrawal of the fee for teaching was wise or not, time will show. I can scarcely forbear, myself, to think that a small fee, five or ten dollars, to be devoted to the maintenance and growth of the medical library, the use of the library being allowed to the students for a small sum held on deposit, to be returned at the end of the session, may yet prove to be the true policy of the Hospital. By this means, a noble medical library might be gathered together, and made useful to the ambitious student. And I am not sure but that the student would value all the more the opportunities given him, and make better use of them, were he to pay a small fee for the privilege.

About the year 1870, it was thought that many of the slighter surgical cases, which had been hitherto kept in the Hospital at a great expense, might be treated as well on the dispensary plan, the patient coming as often as necessary to the Hospital for the proper dressing. Arrangements were made with the staff to try this plan, and the resident physicians on duty in the surgical wards were instructed to dress such cases properly, make any necessary prescription, and direct the patient to return to the house at the time proper to have the treatment carried on. This plan was not yet extended to medical cases. In 1870, about 39 patients were treated in this way per month.

In 1871, the number of out-door patients, medical and surgical, had risen to 594. In 1872, the number reached 663. In the Report for 1873, it appears that this system of out-door relief had become much more important. It is not a true dispensary system, as the Hospital does not furnish medicines to the sick, but limits its work to supplying the proper surgical dressings to surgical cases, and medical advice and prescriptions to the medical cases. Another part of the work, and one that can be made very advantageous to both the sick and the Hospital, is the selection, for admission to the house, of such cases as are specially in need of Hospital aid. Cases thus selected are finally received, or not, as the physician and surgeon on duty may determine.

During the year ending April, 1873, in consequence of the rapid growth of this plan of out-door relief, the work had fallen rather heavily on the resident physicians, so much so as to interfere with their regular in-door duties, and the Managers, therefore, determined to organize a separate staff for the new department. They accordingly elected seven physicians, four of whom were surgeons, to take charge of this department. One physician and one surgeon was to be on duty each day, except Sunday, at a certain hour, to prescribe for all who might apply. Two rooms, those to the north of the gate-way in Eighth Street, were assigned to this purpose. During the year, the number of applicants had risen to 1555, of which 1230 were surgical, and 325 medical.

This department of the city Hospital now grew rapidly, showing clearly the need there was in the city for increased accommodation for the sick poor.

In the Report for 1875, the number of medical cases applying was 619, requiring from the patients 1204 visits; that of surgical cases was 1854, requiring 9750 visits. In all 10,954 visits. The original object of this department was the relief it would afford the Hospital from the maintenance within its wards, at a great expense, of slight or non-dangerous surgical cases, and of mild and chronic medical cases. This class of cases could very well be maintained at home, whilst receiving at the Hospital, as often as might be necessary, the proper advice or dressing for the particular case. But the department was growing rapidly; cases of eye and ear disease, of eruptive disease, as well as those already referred to, were gradually increasing, and the accommodations had become quite inadequate as to space, and most imperfect as to arrangement, though the Managers had, in 1874, built at a cost of under $1000, a new one-story room attached to the building already in use.

The Report for 1876 showed that the whole number of new patients prescribed for had risen to 2975, and the whole number of visits to the Hospital, medical and surgical, to 13,112. At the meeting of the contributors held in May, 1876, a resolution was passed "that the incoming Board be requested to take such measures as they may deem expedient for immediately carrying out the proposed plan for enlarging the accommodations for the treatment of out-door patients." Under this resolution the Board has had plans drawn, not yet formally adopted, which contemplate the erection of a new building, to take the place of the present northeastern house (the north house, as it has been called by the Hospital family). The new building is to be partly on the site of the old one; it is to be made large and roomy, and is expected to contain all the modern improvements necessary for convenience and healthfulness.

The Managers make an earnest appeal to the contributors and to the public for funds to carry out this important object.

Besides the out-door department, the Hospital has arranged a new ward, which has added much to the comfort of the patients. This is the recent-accident ward, which was begun in 1873. A large room on the ground-floor of the north house, close to the main entrance, was chosen for this purpose. Formerly, such cases were taken at all hours of the day or night into the large wards of the house. It requires but little imagination to conceive what must be the confusion in one of these wards, when some severe railroad accident or gunshot wound is suddenly introduced into it, especially in the hours of the night. Let any reader of this history, who has never had a thought of what might be the character of hospital scenes, imagine a dangerous surgical injury—the laceration of a limb, or fracture with the bones driven through the soft parts—bleeding, the waiting and affrighted friends, in whom, probably, pity, as Dr. John Brown says, still remains in large measure a mere emotion, prompting to gesticulations and tears, not having been reasoned and practised into a motive, as it has been in the surgeon and physician. Let him suppose the patient to be one of those unhappy victims to strong drink, who has met his accident in the midst of indulgence; let him imagine the confusion, the noise, the oaths perhaps; let him see, as I have seen, the injured man, waving a broken arm in his drunkenness, or in a fit of mania-a-potu, about his head, making the point of fracture a new centre of motion. It was to avoid such scenes as these that the recent-accident ward was arranged, and the Managers are even now, as was explained above in my history of the out-door department, applying to the public for funds to erect a new building near the entrance, one of the features of which is to afford proper accommodation for such cases.

The Pathological Museum deserves notice, as it is of considerable importance in the system of clinical teaching. In the Report for 1861, I first find the office of pathologist and curator mentioned. The Museum was located at that time in the building on Spruce Street, now occupied by the Historical Society. In 1869, when the new lecture-room was opened for use, the Museum was transferred, as already mentioned, to the basement-room of that building, where it remains to the present day. Under the care of several gentlemen, this Museum has become really valuable. It contains 747 specimens of different morbid preparations, from cases occurring in the house, and may be made of great use in illustrating the medical teaching of the Hospital. In 1875, a course of lectures on Pathological Anatomy, the only one in the city, was given by the pathologist and curator of the Hospital. This course was illustrated by specimens in the Museum.

In 1869, the Managers, anxious to lend all possible

aid to the medical staff in their system of clinical instruction, appointed a new medical officer, under the title of microscopist, whose duty it is to examine any specimen of morbid anatomy, or diseased excretions of the sick, sent to him by the members of the staff on duty. The arrangement has proved wise and useful, particularly for the aid it gives in the diagnosis of disease.

The medical library, after growing rapidly for many years, by the use of the income derived from the small fee charged the students (which had been voluntarily tendered for this purpose by the medical staff), has been but little increased in size, since the lectures were made free in 1871-72. What may be the future condition of this valuable collection of books, we cannot now see. As our cities grow larger, and their schools, colleges, and universities increase in number and extent, the opportunities for study grow apace. For many years, the Hospital library was much the largest and best in the city. Within a few years, however, the demands made upon it have not been so frequent nor so urgent, for the reason that the library of the College of Physicians has come into much greater prominence, under the fostering care of that useful body.

In 1876, the Managers inaugurated for the department of the sick and wounded a plan which had already been introduced into the Insane Department. This was the institution of a system of free beds for the poor. Any one, by a gift to the Hospital of the sum of five thousand dollars, secured a bed in the

Hospital always to be occupied by a poor patient. The average time of stay of patients in the house is about thirty days, so that each free bed will support annually, and send forth to life and work again, or tend and comfort during their last days, some twelve poor patients, who might otherwise have to endure their illness, or end their lives, amidst the keen stings and neglect of poverty and misery. Little do many of the rich know of the wants of the poor. How often have I myself, when on duty at the Hospital, been forced to turn away from the Hospital gate, some forlorn and destitute sick man, or woman, or half-grown youth, who sometimes has added unwilling tears to the appeal already made by his sickness and poverty. Frequently every free bed in the medical wards is full. Not infrequently, we have several over the proper number. The Hospital has, for many years, spent more than its income in the support of this department—what can we—the Managers and the staff—do, but what we have been doing for so many years, cry, give, give. Let me say again that these free beds are noble charities. For five thousand dollars to secure the support, and medical or surgical treatment of twelve poor sick annually forever! What better use could he who has it to give, make of such a sum? For a century and a quarter has this Hospital been in busy operation. It has grown great from feeble beginnings, and has never been suspected of the improper use of money given to it by the charitable.

There are now two free beds attached to this department, one the William A. Blanchard free bed, the money for which was given by Maria E. Blanchard, to perpetuate the memory of her husband. The other is the Warwick Bamfylde Freeman free bed, endowed by Eliza Freeman as a memorial of her son. May we not hope that more of those who have had rare opportunities granted them by Providence for the accumulation of money, may be inspired to give or bequeath of their abundance to the "distempered poor," who are to be always with us?

After these long but necessary details of the history of the department for the sick and wounded, I pass on to that of the department for the insane.

In the year 1851, when Dr. Wood closed his history of the first century of the Hospital, the new department for the insane was already in operation in West Philadelphia. The time had arrived, when it was absolutely necessary, in order to carry out the charter of the institution, to provide new and better accommodations for the insane patients. No longer, under the growing light of modern science, could they be cooped up in the narrow quarters of the town Hospital. It is now well understood by the medical body, and by many of the public, that disease of the mind is not to be cured by mere drugs, nor by that species of solitary confinement to which the insane had hitherto been relegated. Removal from the turmoil of common life, a sense of kind but positive control, agreeable sights and sounds, cheerful company, society, wholesome amusement and occupation, had been found to be the true medicines for insanity;

and they must be obtained for its insane department, if the Pennsylvania Hospital was to continue one of the great charitable institutions of the land.

The purchase by the Managers of the beautiful and valuable property, on which the insane department is located, had been effected in 1836 under the authority of the contributors, and in 1851, when my history of the institution begins, one of the chief buildings, the department for females, had been finished and occupied for just ten years. This property lies, I may say in a few words, about two miles to the west of the Schuylkill River, and, though it was when purchased, an ordinary farm quite out of the town, it is now overlapped by the rapidly growing city at several points, and has graded and paved streets, busy with travel and traffic, passing by its wall. It contains 113 acres, and is becoming constantly a more valuable property, as time moves on. "The Association of Medical Superintendents of American Institutes for the Insane," at their meeting in Philadelphia, 1851, adopted a number of propositions, and ordered them printed in the medical journals of the continent, as the sentiments of the Association. The first proposition asserts that "every hospital for the insane should be in the country, not within less than two miles of a large town, and easily accessible at all seasons." The second proposition asserts that "no hospital for the insane, however limited its capacity, should have less than fifty acres of land, devoted to gardens and pleasure-grounds for its patients. At least one hundred acres should be possessed by every

State hospital, or other institution for two hundred patients, to which number these propositions apply, unless otherwise mentioned."

These propositions reflect the opinions of a body of men of the highest authority in the matter to which they speak, and they point to what must happen in the future to the Pennsylvania Hospital for the Insane. When the time arrives, at which this department shall be compelled by the pressure of the growing city to leave its present location, there can be little doubt that the land will have become so valuable as readily to pay the expenses of removal, erection of new buildings, and, at the same time, increase the capital fund of the Hospital.

In 1851, ten years after its opening, the Hospital was inconveniently crowded, though the Report states that "the general good health which then prevailed, enabled us to receive all the cases that were brought to the Hospital, although much difficulty was often experienced in accommodating them." In 1852, "notwithstanding the extensive provision for the insane made by the State at Harrisburg, and which has been available during the year just closed, this institution has been about full during the whole period, and for much of the time inconveniently crowded, particularly in the ward appropriated to men." In the Report for 1853, it appears again that "during the entire year, the institution has been rather more than comfortably filled, the average number for the whole period, as shown above, being 229, while 220 is regarded as the capacity of the building.

Anxious to receive all who desired admission, we have at no previous time refused any suitable applicant; but during a part of the year just closed, we were for a time compelled, although with great reluctance, to decline receiving patients, except under the most urgent circumstances."

In the Report for 1853, it is stated that "Pennsylvania has within its limits, at this day, not less than 2500 insane, and hospital accommodations for only 930."

After travelling carefully over the whole ground, the physician-in-chief, Dr. Kirkbride, distinctly recommends an extension by the Pennsylvania Hospital of its accommodations for the insane. He opposes any material extension of the very large and handsome building on the ground, deeming it unwise to have more than 200, or 250 at the outside, in one building. He thinks "it important for the best interests of the afflicted that the increased accommodations that are required for the insane should be provided under the auspices of that noble charity, which, more than a century ago, began the great work in America, and which has ever since conducted its important trust in a manner to command the confidence of the whole community."

An entirely new building for 200 male patients was proposed—to be placed on the seventy acres of land then comprising the farm of the institution, while the existing building, with everything included within the external wall, should be given up for the exclusive use of as many females. This tract of land could be readily inclosed; it had two fine groves of forest trees, and a never-failing spring of good water, and remarkable facilities for draining. Dr. Kirkbride knows of no benefit from the presence of the two sexes in one building, sees several advantages in separate buildings, as greater liberty for all the patients, more privacy, and more extended use of the most valuable means of treatment. He believes that the funds necessary for the new building can be obtained from the benevolent citizens of Philadelphia.

In the Report for 1854, it appears that the Hospital, during this year, had been always full, and frequently much crowded. All suitable applicants were received, when the state of the house would justify their reception, "but during a few months of the summer and autumn, our numbers were so large, and the tendency to sickness in the community in general so great, that, in justice to the patients already with us, we felt compelled to decline a large part of those who applied for admission. During this period, as many as fifty individuals laboring under mental diseases, and in every way proper cases for care and treatment in such an institution, and who would have been glad to avail themselves of our accommodations, were compelled to look elsewhere for relief." With this fact in mind, and reflecting, too, that insanity spares no class, no age, no sex, no calling; that Pennsylvania, with between 2500 and 3000 insane within her limits, has accommodation for but 930; that Philadelphia and the adjacent country, with certainly more than 1200 insane, has accommodation for only 630; that diseases of the mind, to be treated with every chance of success, must be treated in the early stages; considering the terrible strain upon a household, to which the care of an insane person falls—the anxiety, suffering, the possible injury to others; Dr. Kirkbride repeats and urges with great force the recommendation of the previous year, for a further extension of the usefulness of the Hospital.

He reasons that, if 400, instead of 200, insane are provided for, from eighty to one hundred will annually be restored to reason and usefulness in society, and that many others will be greatly improved, while the whole community will be protected from the dangerous acts of irresponsible men. He states, also, that thirty or forty poor could be maintained on the free list, and between sixty and seventy others, in moderate circumstances, be taken care of at a rate of board considerably below the actual cost of their support.

In 1855, the same overcrowding of the wards continued, and more than fifty applicants were again, literally for want of space, refused.

In 1853, after Dr. Kirkbride's first recommendation for an extension of the Hospital, to take the form of an entirely new building, with separation of the sexes, the Managers, having approved the plan, submitted it to the contributors, who also approved, and appointed a committee to aid the Board in procuring the necessary subscriptions.

On May 1, 1854, the Managers issued an "Appeal

to the citizens of Pennsylvania for means to provide additional accommodations for the insane." This appeal was afterwards, by resolution of the Board, printed as an appendix to the fifteenth Annual Report of the Pennsylvania Hospital for the insane.

The appeal recites the facts that this Hospital, which, since its foundation in 1751, had already received in its wards 58,600 patients, of whom 33,900 had been on the free list, was emphatically the fruit of the charity of the people of Philadelphia, and of the State of Pennsylvania, all the work just cited having been effected without assistance from city, county, or the State, with the exception of certain small appropriations made by the Provincial Assembly, and by the State legislature towards the close of the last century, and which latter sum had been expended in the erection of the original building in the city of Philadelphia. The appeal shows that the Hospital authorities have been compelled, for some years past, to listen "to the urgent entreaties almost daily made for accommodations which do not exist;" it recites the fact that insanity, to be successfully treated, must be treated early, and that, therefore, cases thus deferred by necessity, grow more and more hopeless; it argues that insanity is much more successfully treated, as a rule, in hospitals specially adapted to the purpose, than at home; and reasserts the now well-proved fact that "the present institutions are more than full, the demands for admission are steadily increasing, and additional buildings must be promptly provided, or great loss and suffering must soon result to the community." It goes on to say that, in order to meet these demands, "a plan has recently been proposed by the physician of the Hospital for the insane, after a careful study of the whole subject, which meets the entire approbation of this Board, which they cordially commend to the sympathy of the whole community, and to carry out which thoroughly, they now make this earnest appeal to their fellow-citizens." The appeal states that a sum of $250,000 will be required to carry out the object, and that the payment of no contribution will be asked for, until at least $150,000 shall have been subscribed. They propose, also, to perpetuate the memory of any one who shall subscribe $10,000, by naming one of the wards, into which the Hospital will be divided, after the donor; and also that the gift of $5000 shall be considered as securing forever one free bed.

Up to the spring of 1855, more than $127,000 had been subscribed, and the Managers were determined to begin the work, so soon as the sum of $150,000 should be reached.

In the spring of 1856, the subscriptions had reached the sum of $209,000, of which amount, however, sixteen subscribers of $1000 each conditioned their gift on the basis that the whole sum, $250,000, should be raised before the close of the year 1857.

The new building was begun on the 7th July, 1856, and was opened for the reception of patients on the 27th of October, 1859.

"It is situated," says the Report, "in full view and on the western side of the buildings previously in use, at a distance in a right line of 648 yards, and in the midst of fifty acres of pleasure-grounds and gardens, the whole of which are surrounded by a substantial stone-wall, covered with flagging, and of an average height of ten and a half feet. The gate of entrance is on Forty-ninth Street (an avenue intended to be 100 feet wide), between Market and Haverford Streets, and by each of which, by means of horse railroads, easy access to Forty-ninth Street can be had at all seasons.

"This new Hospital faces the west, and consists of a centre building, with wings running north and south, making a front of 512 feet; of other wings, connected with each of those just referred to, running east a distance of 167 feet, all three stories high, and these last having at their extreme ends communications with extensive one-storied buildings. All the exterior walls are of stone, stuccoed, and the interior are of brick.

"This arrangement gives provision for the accommodation of sixteen distinct classes of male patients in the new building, as the same number of classes of females are now provided for in that previously in use. Each of these sixteen wards has connected with it, besides the corridors for promenading and the chambers of the patients and attendants, a parlor, a dining-room, a bath-room, a water-closet, a urinal, a sink-room, a wash-room, a drying-closet, a storeroom for brushes and buckets, a clothes-room, a dumbwaiter, a dust-flue, and a stairway passing out of doors, if desired, without communication with the other wards; and every room in the building, almost without exception, has a flue communicating with the fresh air duct, for warm or cool air, according to the season (and hereafter to be referred to), and with the main ventilating trunks which terminate in the various ventilators on the roof of the building.

"The centre building is 115 by 73 feet. It has a handsome doric portico of granite in front, and is surmounted by a dome of good proportions, in which are placed the iron tanks from which the whole building is supplied with water. The lantern on the dome is 119 feet from the pavement, and from it is a beautiful panoramic view of the fertile and highly improved surrounding country, the Delaware and Schuylkill Rivers, and the city of Philadelphia, with its many prominent objects of interest."

The new building had cost, with its various fixtures and arrangements, up to 1859, $322,542.86, and $30,000 additional were required to meet other liabilities that had been incurred.

It is impossible for me—I have not the space—to describe in detail the various interesting points connected with the internal arrangements, the housekeeping—so to speak—of the new Hospital.

Of all the matters connected with the domestic arrangements of a hospital, nothing is more important than the heating and ventilation. To supply to each person so many cubic feet of fresh air per hour, winter and summer, has been long one of the problems over which medical men, architects, builders, and housekeepers have puzzled. The new building is ventilated by a fan, driven by steam. The fan is of cast iron, with an extreme diameter of 16 feet, and a width of 4 feet. It makes from 30 to 60 revolutions per minute, as may be required. The fresh air passing to the fan, is received from a tower, 40 feet high, so that all surface exhalations are avoided. The air is then driven through a duct, $8\frac{1}{2}$ by $10\frac{1}{2}$ feet at the mouth, into all parts, distant as well as near, of the building. "From this cold-air duct, openings lead into the different warm-air chambers, which in the one-storied buildings are covered with slate; but, in all other parts of the Hospital, these chambers and air-ducts are arched with brick, laid with smooth joints. The warm air, in nearly all cases, is admitted near the floor, and the ventilators open near the ceiling, always in the interior corridor" walls. The different ventilating flues terminate in the attic in close ducts, either of brick or wood, smoothly plastered, increasing in size about thirty per cent. more rapidly than the capacity of the flues entering them, by which, through the different belvideres on the roof, they communicate with the external atmosphere. In the centre-building, the ventilation is through the dome.

Besides the fan, there is another feature in the method of ventilation which I must refer to. The gases from the boiler enter a common flue, which passes on to an underground flue, four feet wide and six feet high, a distance of 557 feet, ascending 31 feet in its course, till it comes to the foot of the main chimney, which rises to a height of 78 feet above the surface of the ground. The chimney is six feet in diameter from bottom to top, and it is made the ventilating power for securing a strong downward draft of air through all the water closets, urinals, sinks, and bath-tubs in the entire establishment. It is placed, therefore, in a central position on the eastern side of the building.

What could be more perfect than this? In the original plans for the building all these points had been provided for. The cellar was dug and proportioned, the foundation walls laid, the different stories built, and the floors and walls pierced, as they were under the workmen's hands, by the ducts, passages, and flues necessary for this magnificent system of ventilation. I doubt whether there is in the United States, a public building more admirably adapted for its purposes, than this department for the males of the Pennsylvania Hospital for the Insane.

The building is heated entirely by steam. No fire is used in any part of it for heating purposes, though open fireplaces have been introduced into all the parlors and many of the large rooms, in case they should be needed. The only fires inside its walls are those in the kitchen, bake-, and ironing-rooms. The boilers for the generation of steam are in the engine-room, which is placed 71 feet beyond the nearest point of the Hospital building, thus avoiding all danger of fire to the main building, much of the danger of explosion, which, though so improbable, must be considered, and all noise, dust, and other small inconveniences. The steam is carried from the boilers by a five-inch welded iron pipe to the cellar of the Hospital building, and is there distributed into eighty-three air-chambers, from which direct flues lead into the apartments above.

I might, had I time, say a great deal more upon many interesting points—about the water-supply, obtained from large springs within the grounds, and, of late, by a direct communication with the city water works; of the powerful steam-pumps, capable of raising 10,000 gallons per hour, and of the water-tanks in the dome, which hold 21,000 gallons. I might describe the carpenter shop, the carriage house and stables, the patients' rooms, the window and corridor-guards, the stairways, most of which are fire-proof, the sewerage, which is admirable, the bath-rooms and water-closets, of which there are twenty-one in the building, beside those in the patients' rooms, the lighting, furniture, cooking and distribution of food, the provision against fire, the laundry arrangements, the pleasure-gardens, and a number of other things, but must refer the reader who wishes to have a clear understanding of the great amount of thought and intelligence, necessary to take care of a family of 250 insane persons, to the reports of the physician-in-chief, and especially to the Report for the year 1859. Let any one study these reports, and then reflect upon the extent, variety, and minuteness of the provision made, and I am sure he will not cavil about the expensiveness of a great hospital, but will see for himself that expense is unavoidable.

Occasionally, an outcry has been raised against what the objectors have been pleased to call "palaces for the insane." What would these critics have? A building to contain from 200 to 250 patients, with officers, attendants, cooks, bakers; with offices, sitting-rooms, bed-rooms, bath-rooms, water-closets, ironing-rooms, and kitchens; can such a building be other than large and imposing? Is it a palace, simply because it is vast? This element of size cannot be avoided, and the question reduces itself to the simple alternative, Shall the so-called palace be imposing by the hugeness of its deformity, or by fitness for its purposes, and by the beauty of its outlines?

But such cavils against insane hospitals come only from the thoughtless. I have always felt, and shall always feel, grateful to the Managers of this Hospital, for the fine taste they have shown in the style and architecture of these buildings. Amongst the pious uses of money is the embellishment of cities. Mr. Binney, in his famous argument for this city in the Girard will case, shows that property was left "*ad pias causas*," or "charitable uses," in the earliest periods of English history. At page 78 of the printed argument he says that "charitable uses were settled at common law long before the earliest of these dates (1307, 1334, 1377), and, doubtless, from the first dawn of Christianity." He adds: "Any person who was an object of compassion, an orphan, widow, or pauper, destitute of support from himself, those rendered infirm by disease or age, being also poor—the watching of a city, the repairing of bridges, walls, and

4

ditches of a city or castle; the ornaments and fabrics of churches; lights, anniversaries, and incidents relating to divine worship; these were all included under *piæ causæ.*" In the opening of his argument before the Supreme Court, he makes use of this idea of the embellishment of our city, as one of the chief grounds on which he claims the judgment and sympathy of the court, for he declares that the complainants against the city "now claim the decree of this Court to defeat the great purpose of his (Girard's) life," . . . . . "to frustrate the two nearest and dearest wishes of his heart, and the two noblest objects upon earth that, living or dying, can fill the heart of any man, the instruction and succor of the fatherless poor, and the security, comfort, and embellishment of a great city." Observe how Mr. Binney puts the case before the grand and august body he is addressing—the two noblest objects a man can have, charity to the poor and needy, and the security, comfort, and embellishment of a great city.

We cannot be too thankful that the buildings for the insane were made handsome, striking, and picturesque. Some one of these cavillers, or any one of us, may yet have to place in an insane asylum some one near and dear to us. Who knows what the morrow shall bring forth? If it were to be so, should we choose a building with the air of a prison, penitentiary, or great uncouth and rambling hotel, or a well-proportioned, attractive, and imposing house for the poor afflicted one to dwell in?

No, for one, I rejoice in these handsome and attractive buildings for the insane. I think it must be only a weak, pitiful mind, and a cruel soul, that would refuse to these afflicted ones such sweet pleasures of the senses as we may be able to give them.

The next step taken by the Managers was the repair and improvement of the original building, which had now become the department for females. It had been in constant use for nineteen years, and had been all the time so full that but few repairs could be undertaken. It was thoroughly repaired. The heating apparatus was overhauled, all the water-fixtures, bath-rooms, and water-closets were put in complete order, often by an entire renewal of the fixtures; one new bath-room and six new water-closets were introduced, and a great deal more was done which I cannot particularize. Two new and fine rooms were arranged, one to be used as a reception ward, and the other as a sewing ward, for the use of the patients. The lecture-room was elegantly and newly fitted up by a friend to the Hospital. This work was done in the year 1860, and cost about $25,000.

In 1866, reference is made to the necessity for a new ward at the women's department. In 1867, this additional ward was in process of erection. It was intended for "a class of cases of the deepest interest— for persons very sick, and for those laboring under acute affections of the brain, accompanied by high excitement, and requiring the utmost care and privacy, and yet, for obvious reasons, not comfortably situated in any of the ordinary wards." This had been admirably provided for in the new department, that for males, but not in that for females. As the wards of the latter became full, the necessity for extra accommodations for this class of cases became more and more apparent. About this time, a benevolent citizen of Philadelphia, a childless man and unmarried, Joseph Fisher, left by will to the contributors of the Pennsylvania Hospital one-half of the residue of his estate " to be devoted to extending and improving the accommodations for the insane." The total amount received by the Hospital was $57,511.57. He died in 1862.

The new building was commenced in 1867, and finished in 1868. It was opened for use in December, 1868, and was called the "Fisher Ward." Some years later, in 1873, when a second building of the same kind was erected, from the funds of the same estate, the former was called the "South Fisher Ward," and the latter the "North Fisher Ward."

The South Fisher Ward is placed on the south side of the large yard, belonging to the third south ward, and connects with the eighth ward, on the south side of the Hospital, by a passage taken from the drying-room. The building is 112 feet long, by $27\frac{1}{2}$ feet wide, and has two stories, each 12 feet in height. It is built of brick, is stuccoed, and has a slate roof. The connection with the eighth ward is fire-proof. The North Fisher Ward is on the east side of the North fifth ward, with which it is connected by a light and airy vestibule $11\frac{1}{2}$ by $8\frac{1}{2}$ feet, and through which access may be had to the new ward, without going through any part of the Hospital. This building is 125 by 40 feet, and has two stories, each 12 feet high. It is built of brick, above the foundation-walls, which are of stone. All the brick walls are hollow, an airspace being left between the outer and inner portions.

The internal arrangements of these wards are perfect. It is impossible for me to describe them in detail; but let any one who may read this history examine for himself, and he will say that few private houses have such conveniences. The South Fisher Ward has, on the first floor, besides bath-rooms, water-closets, and clothes-closets, nine rooms for patients, each about 10 by $14\frac{1}{2}$ feet; in a few instances, two are thrown together. The rooms are on one side of a corridor, partly $8\frac{1}{2}$, and partly $10\frac{1}{2}$ feet wide, and with two bay-windows projecting more than four feet, in each story. The second story has very nearly the same arrangement. All the patients' rooms have a cheerful southern exposure, with large windows, the upper sashes of which are of iron, immovable, while the lower are of wood, and may be raised to their full height, having ornamental wrought-iron guards on the outside. The windows all have Venetian shutters.

The North Fisher Ward has two stories, with rooms on both sides of a corridor 12 feet wide; it has large bay-windows at either end, and another in an alcove or parlor 12 feet by 20, on the south side. These bay-windows light the corridors admirably well. Each of the two stories is so arranged that it may be divided, for the sake of quiet and privacy, into three sections, by means of sliding doors, which have ground glass in their panels. The size of the patients' rooms varies from 9 by 11 to 13 by 11 feet, and some of them are connected. In each alcove is placed a piano, and in each bay-window a cottage organ.

The heating and ventilating arrangements for these two wards are on the same general plan as those of the department for males. Great attention was paid, during the erection of the buildings, to these points. The heating is by steam, and the ventilation by a fan. The air, after being warmed by contact with the steam radiators, passes into flues, all of which, both for heat and ventilation, are in the interior corridor walls, completely filling them. They are made of very smooth terra cotta, with rounded corners, each 3 by 13 inches, and are placed in the centre of the walls. The warm air is admitted near the floor into every room, and in numerous places in the corridors. The ventilating flues, corresponding with the heating in number and size, have openings invariably near the floor, and also near the ceiling, all of which can be controlled by keys provided for the purpose. The air passes through these ventilating flues into the attic, the whole of which in the middle of the building—12 feet wide—is a foul air-duct, with a division through its centre, so as to prevent any interference with currents from opposite sides. The foul air is finally carried off into chimneys having an ascending current of heated air. The water-closets all have a downward draft, connecting with these chimneys.

The South Fisher Ward cost $24,850; the North Fisher Ward building cost $31,250.01, its heating and ventilation, water, and gas arrangements $8207.62. and its furniture $3831.49.

I have now traced the history of the Insane Department from 1851 to 1873, when it stood before the world much as it stands now, an institution with two expensive and very handsome buildings, situated on a fine landed property of 113 acres, on the edge of one of the great cities of America, and close to a park of 2700 acres, which I have heard called by a travelled gentleman of great taste and experience "the finest rural drive in the world." These two large buildings, with their annexes, afford room, each, for 250 patients. In 1875, the total number of patients was 684. The highest number at any one time was 450, the lowest 406, and the average number during the whole period was 430; 208 males, and 222 females.

And the wonder of it! that this fine estate should have been bought, and the noble buildings which adorn it, erected, without state or government aid of any kind. Except that the Provincial Assembly of Pennsylvania voted a small sum in 1751, and that the Assembly gave, at the close of the last century, about seventy thousand dollars for the erection of the city buildings, the Hospital has had no aid from state or city government. It has lived and grown great upon the free gifts of the citizens of Philadelphia and Pennsylvania.

The land was purchased—as has been told by Dr. Wood—in 1836, for 30,000 dollars. This money, and the cost of the first building erected—that which is now the department for females—was obtained by the sale of open lots around the city hospital, which had been purchased by the Managers many years before at a very low price. Soon after the opening of the Insane Department, it became overcrowded, as I have already told, and it was plainly necessary either to restrict the admissions, or to increase the accommodations.

Once again, in 1866, it became necessary to erect some new wards for the Female Department. The accommodations for a certain class of patients were not so good in the department for females as in that for males, as the latter had been planned and built after all the experience gained for years in the former. It was, therefore, thought necessary to have some additional and better accommodations for this class of cases. Out of this arose the two beautiful, most complete, and perfect wards for this end that I can imagine—the Fisher wards.

I have to advert next to some of the interior concerns of the Hospital, some of which are of purely medical, and some of general public interest. I refer specially to the provision made for the comfort, happiness, and cure of the patients. An insane hospital differs from all others in one important point: few of the patients pass less than several months inside its walls, and many are destined to pass years, or even the greater part of a lifetime, within these narrow limits; were nothing done for the occupation and recreation of these unfortunates, their home would be little better than a jail. But this is not all. Their cure depends largely upon the moral treatment brought to bear upon them.

The reports from year to year demonstrate that not drugs alone, and a life such as is led in hospitals for the sick, will suffice for the insane. It is plain that, to cure the curable and comfort the incurable, there must be supplied to the patients fresh air, exercise, occupation, and amusement. These things, which the healthy child or man makes for himself as naturally as the bird sings, the ant toils, and the kids skip upon the hills, it becomes the duty of the medical authorities of an insane hospital to supply to its inmates. From the earliest period of Dr. Kirkbride's connection with the Hospital, he has been toiling in this direction. In the earlier reports, these matters are treated under the head of the Farm and Garden, Workshop and Mechanical Department, Ward Libraries, Museum, and Reading Rooms, as in 1852; in the later reports, they are described under the title of "Evening Entertainments, Occupation, and Amusement of the Patients."

In 1853, it is related that the ninth course of lectures and evening entertainments is now in progress.

In 1866, the Report says, "the importance of evening entertainments, as now conducted here, can hardly be overestimated. The long experience we have had has only tended to confirm this conviction, and each year we have been able to add something that tended to increase their attractiveness and efficacy. For the first time, I am able to report that at the Department for Females, every evening in the week is now provided with some means of breaking up the monotony of the wards, formerly so universal in institutions for the insane. It is not many years since the condition of the patients, in their badly lighted halls, without any means of passing the dreary hours that came upon them every day between their evening meal and bedtime, was certainly one of the saddest sights witnessed in too many of these establishments. In this Hospital, of the seven evenings of the week, for nine months of the year, one is now devoted to reading of the Bible and sacred music, three to lectures, exhibition of dissolving views with music, or concerts, in the lecture-room, two to light gymnastic exercises with music in the new hall put up expressly for that purpose, and one to tea parties in the resident officers' department, and at which all the officers are generally present. These last are composed of as many patients as the dining-room will accommodate, and the officers' weekly parties have now become one of the regular means of passing our evenings. Care is taken, as far as possible, to invite those who will be most likely to enjoy each other's society, and it has been found that there was no ward that was not able to take its turn in these pleasant reunions. Even of those from the most excited wards, and of the most chronic class of patients, there have been few that were not able to participate, and the enjoyment of those for whom this provision was made, has very rarely, if ever, been diminished by any unpleasant occurrence."

I have made this long extract, in the words of the Report, that the reader might see for himself how important, as a means of treatment, the recreation and amusements of the patients have become in this Hospital. I will pause for a moment to ask whether these experiences of an intelligent medical observer, of the value of amusements for the solace and cure of the insane, ought not to lead us to a higher appreciation of their value for the well. Are not the Germans, as a nation, wiser than we, in the national habit they have formed of giving more of their time to entertainment and relaxation? They do no less work than we, of all kinds, mental and muscular, and yet appear to suffer less from insanity.

In the Report for 1858, will be found a list of the subjects treated at no less than 122 of these evening lectures, and any one, who will take the trouble to glance at the list, will be surprised, I am sure, at its extent and variety, and yet more surprised to know that the hard-working assistant medical officers of the house, were the authors of much the larger part. Surely, the post of assistant physician in the insane department of this Hospital has been no sinecure.

A like system of evening entertainments, with slight differences, is carried out in the department for males.

Besides the resources just mentioned for the wholesome occupation and amusement of the patients in the evenings, other analogous means are employed as amongst the most valuable influences in the medical and moral treatment of the disease.

Fresh air is insisted upon by means of walks once, and, in proper cases, twice, a day in the beautiful grounds of the institution, which have been so arranged that, within the ninety-one acres that are inclosed, there are nearly four miles of dry walks and drives. The Hospital keeps, moreover, all the carriages it can afford, and donkeys and ponies, and every day that will allow all these means of locomotion are put into use. Let no one suppose that there is extravagance in this. All this apparatus belongs to the methods of cure, and a large part of it consists of free gifts. It is touching to read, year after year, the acknowledgments to kind friends of the Hospital for a horse for the use of the patients; for the loan of a horse; for a second-hand carriage; for a pony, for a donkey for the use of the patients; for money to fit up the lecture-room; and for money to build a new reading-room. Many, indeed most, of the special means of occupation I have referred to, are the fruit of numerous small gifts from many different hands. The gardens, both vegetable and flower, the workshop and mechanical department, the lawns, the walks, the roads, the calisthenics, each for its proper cases and sex, are employed to secure that muscular work which is known to be so valuable an aid in the treatment of nervous diseases. In 1864, there was erected by the "generous liberality of our friends, for the special benefit and amusement of the patients" a new building, called the Gymnastic Hall, near the north return wing of the Department for Females. This hall could not have been built from the ordinary resources of the Hospital, but, as has often happened, when the need was known, friends came forward and supplied the money for the special purpose. The building is 51 by 32 feet in the inside, with a ceiling 17 feet high. There are two corridors of good size, the floor is double, and the hall is well arranged for heating and lighting. It contains an excellent piano and a fine melodeon. Comfortable seats are provided for about one hundred and thirty persons, while the portion of the floor specially devoted to the exercises is 40 by 17 feet. A system of light gymnastics had been introduced under a proper teacher, and it is pleasing to observe, from year to year, the great interest felt by the patients in this, to them, unsuspected method of treatment. In 1866, they had been continued for three years, and the interest in them was undiminished. The class exercising averaged between twenty and thirty, and the number of spectators was considerable. In the Report for 1875, we read that the "light gymnastics, for which the hall bearing that name was specially provided, have been continued regularly for eleven years, with undiminished interest and usefulness." Let me repeat that this constant attention to what might seem to be a mere system of amusements, constitutes one of the most potent means of medical treatment. They are as purely medical as Ling's movement cure, or the regular exercises to the sound of a fife and drum, carried out, under a polytechnic professor, at the Children's Hospital in Paris. They are as truly scientific medical means as is the prescription of a New York, Philadelphia, or London doctor, to a broken-down banker, broker, or professional man, with his brain-fag, to go to Lake Superior, to the Adirondacks, or to the Continent, or the South of Europe.

No one, who has not visited with intelligent care, and more than once in his life, an insane hospital, or who has not devoted some time to a study of the reports of such hospitals, can conceive of the multitude and variety of arrangements necessary for the proper care and medical treatment of the patients.

In the Report for 1861, I find a suggestion in regard to the care of patients, which it is proper to mention. The constant charge, the personal care, the watching, the nursing of the insane, that care which parents give to the helpless child, devolves upon the attendants or nurses. There must be a sufficient number of these to have one, at least, at all times, in each ward with the patients. This rule renders two attendants necessary for each ward, for some patients of each class leave the ward to walk, and for other purposes, and there must be a second attendant for those who remain. More than this may be necessary, as, for instance, when some of the patients are particularly troublesome, dangerous to others, or suicidal. The duties of these nurses are numerous and varied, and one of the luxuries of a hospital is to have as many as can be used with advantage, without restriction by reason of scarcity of funds. It was suggested, therefore, in 1861, that in addition to the ordinary attendants or nurses, there should be another class of persons to be called companions, or, as they have sometimes been designated, teachers. These officers, it was intended, should be able to give their attention wherever specially required, and to devote as much time to individual cases as might be deemed profitable. As they were to have no ordinary ward duties, they could devote themselves to the task of rendering the patients all such services as would tend to make them more contented and happy. It is astonishing, indeed, how the poor insane patient will brighten up and become cheerful for a kind word spoken in season. They, moreover, it was thought, would have a good effect upon the ordinary attendants, for these, knowing that, in addition to the regular visits of the physician and other officers of the house, they were liable to be seen at any moment by the companions or teachers, would be more careful in their conduct towards the patients. Accordingly, in 1869, I find this suggestion in full operation. At "the department for males, there are two supervisors, whose duties are entirely among the patients, while, at the department for females, there are one supervisor and two companions to those under care, who, released from all labor in the wards, devote themselves to the comfort and well-being of the patients, each one making a daily written report to the chief medical officer of the respective departments." It is added in the report that it is in this direction that increased expenditure may be profitably made.

Reference has already been made to the separation of the sexes, at the time when the demands upon the Hospital became so urgent as to render the erection of a new building necessary. Previously to that time, in this, and, I believe, to this day, in most insane hospitals, the sexes were lodged in the same building, either in opposite wings, or, as was the case in the old insane wards of this institution, in the Pine Street Hospital, in different stories of the same wing.

In 1853, in urging the erection of a new building, the physician-in-chief writes: "I know of no benefit resulting from the presence of the two sexes in the same building, and there are various disadvantages. While the separation of the sexes would prove advantageous, the proximity of the two establishments might be made mutually beneficial." As we have already seen, the plan of having a building for each sex was adopted, and it has worked so well that the physician-in chief recommends it as the best, wherever there is room upon the grounds and funds sufficient for the purpose. Among the advantages enumerated are the increase in the liberty of the patients, from the fact that their pleasure grounds, drives, and walks can be doubled in extent, and the fences formerly necessary to divide the grounds be taken away. A much more proper classification, also, of the cases can be made. Where, formerly, there were eight, there are now sixteen classes for each sex. The mental condition of many patients is said to be less troublesome under this arrangement. These, and other facts, induce me to believe that there are, on the whole, many advantages in the separation of the sexes, and none, unless it be economy of space, in favor of the opposite plan.

In the Report for 1875, are some remarks upon

mechanical restraint. The ground is taken that, while every effort should be made to avoid its use as far as possible, no inflexible rule ought to be made against it, but that its use or disuse should be left to the physician-in-chief, who is, after all, the only person really competent to decide the question. Under this rule, its abuse would be avoided, since no mere attendant or inferior officer could, upon his own will or judgment, employ it, while the only person fit to be trusted with such responsible power, would have the right to use it in the few cases where it is the lesser of unavoidable evils. For my own part, I may say that I have seen cases of insanity in private practice, in which enforced confinement to a chair or bed, from time to time, appeared to me essential to save a violent patient from dangerous exhaustion.

Up to the year 1875, the medical duties of this department had been carried on by four physicians, the physician-in-chief, with an assistant physician for the department of females, and two assistant physicians in the other department. In 1875, as the Hospital had had for over two years an average of more than two hundred patients in each department, the number was again increased in accordance with the recommendation of the Association of Superintendents of the Insane. An assistant physician was added to each department, making six in all. This increase of the medical staff will enable the physicians to give more time to the wards, to study the cases thoroughly, to become more familiar with such patients as specially need personal intercourse with, and the moral influence of, a physician, and, lastly, to make scientific records of the great variety of mental diseases constantly in the Hospital.

Having concluded what I have to say in detail of the history of the Hospital, I wish, before closing this imperfect sketch, to make some remarks upon the institution as a whole.

Little could Dr. Thomas Bond, or even that many-sided genius, Franklin, when they began their labors in the cause of this Hospital, foresee to what a height of honor and usefulness the institution would rise in the course of a century and a quarter. Dr. Thomas Bond died in 1784, and Franklin in 1790. They had lived long enough to see the birth of their idea, and its fair progress during the first thirty-odd years of its growth. But no foresight of theirs, either practical or poetic, could have told them that, in one hundred and twenty-five years, this institution would be spending annually, in the care of the sick and wounded, and insane patients, nearly twice as much money as its whole capital at the time of its foundation; and that during this period of time, a century and a quarter, it would have had under its roof no less than 103,074 patients, of which number, 63,899 were indigent poor, who had to be boarded, fed, medicined, and not a few, partially at least, clothed. Now the Hospital has three large and noble buildings to receive its sick; it owns a square of ground in the old city, and 113 acres in the new one beyond the Schuylkill, of the future existence of which Bond and Franklin could have had no more than some vague dream.

It has grown great. It has built great houses, and built them apparently on the rock. It has tended an army of the sick. Could the destitute sick poor, who have passed through its gates without charge, be marshalled into a visible array, we should behold an army greater by three-fold than the largest Washington ever commanded, and only a few thousand less than that with which Wellington arrested at Waterloo the progress of the greatest and most insatiate conqueror of the modern world.

And how has this army been lodged, and fed, and ruled? Under what system of administration has all this been effected? Surely, the organization of so successful a staff as this must be worth some study.

The power—the active energy—in this machine, lies in the Board of Managers. This Board has but one check upon it, the fact that it must be elected annually by the contributors. The contributors represent the latent heat of the machine, which, should it become necessary, may burst into active energy of its own. Once a Manager elected, he serves so long as he serves well, if he will to do so, for the contributors do not believe, fortunately for this army of the poor, in rotation in office, but, the better a Manager does his work of managing, and the longer he has served, the better the contributors like him, and the less they will disturb him. And then—the beauty of it—to this day, he serves without pay. Were he paid, it is to be feared that the poor would be poorer, for then might come rotation in office, and locusts and grasshoppers, who, to exist, would have to appropriate some of the good things provided for the poor.

The Board of Managers, then, is the *vis viva*, the soul, heart, and mind of the Pennsylvania Hospital. It is like the King—it never dies. Composed of twelve men, it has cherished and ruled the Hospital for one hundred and twenty-five years. It elects all the officers but the Treasurer. It collects and spends the money. It is responsible for each and every failure, and for every success. It chooses the medical and surgical staff for the sick and wounded department, and the physician-in-chief and the medical assistants for the insane department. Can any one say that it has not chosen well? Is it not one of the boasts of the Hospital, that it has always furnished to the poor, the best medical and surgical talent to be found in Philadelphia? It has secured for the poor many of the most distinguished medical names of the country, Bond, Cadwalader, Rush, Physick, Norris, Pancoast. But why should I prolong the list? All Philadelphia knows perfectly well that her ablest physicians and surgeons have been glad to serve the Pennsylvania Hospital.

The Board governs the expenditures. It must regulate the expenses by the income, and, when the means do not suffice for the needs of the institution, it has but one resource, the public, not State or city, but the general public. And we have seen already how well this public has been satisfied with the action of the Board, for has it not, in answer to such appeals, given large sums of money?

The Managers superintend the operations of the two departments of the Hospital by means of visiting Committees or visitors. The Board appoints two members of their body on each of these Committees, and the Committees pay regular weekly visits to each branch of the institution. The members of the Committees inspect the wards, see the officers, hear reports, and examine accounts. These duties are now, and always have been performed, with great regularity. This system of visitation and inspection is of essential consequence to both branches; to the insane department, it is vital. The public, from time to time, becomes excited upon all matters connected with hospitals for the insane. Stories are told in sensational novels, and sometimes in the newspapers, or whispered among the credulous and ignorant, of the unjust imprisonment of oppressed citizens in such institutions; and occasionally patients are brought before the courts, by writs of habeas corpus, obtained by friends, who refuse to believe in the fact of insanity.

The only ground for these reports is the fact that, occasionally, in the past, an improper use has been made of insane hospitals. But no such iniquity can be traced to this Hospital, nor, do I believe, to any other in this country. I will quote from the Report for the Insane Department for the year 1872, the opinion of an able and distinguished writer on Medical Jurisprudence. He says: "We have yet to learn of the first well-authenticated case in this country; and we have heard the same thing asserted by others whose professional duties have enabled them to be well informed on this subject. Although this does not prove the impossibility of such an abuse, it certainly does prove that it must be an exceedingly rare occurrence."

The weekly visits by the Managers to the insane department is a duty which the superintendent declares has never been neglected. The State Hospitals for the insane are visited and watched over by officials appointed by the State. In this Hospital this same duty is performed by these Visiting Committees of the Board of Managers.

I have said that the Board has but one check upon it, the fact that it is elected annually by the contributors, but I must add that the Board acts under the original charter granted by the Provincial Assembly. In this charter, are several provisions so excellent that I will cite them for the benefit of the reader. One is that the treasurer is elected by the contributors at the same period, once a year, when they elect the Managers. This gives to the treasurer a higher position on the Hospital staff, than any other officer save the Managers themselves, and invests him with a certain independent responsibility and dignity, which he could not have, were he merely a creation of the Managers. Another provision of the charter, which seems to me admirable, is that in which it is declared "That no general meeting of the said contributors, nor any persons acting under them, shall employ any money or estate, expressly given or added to the capital stock of the said Hospital, in any other way than by applying its annual interest or rent towards the entertainment and care of the sick and distempered poor, that shall be from time to time brought and placed therein for the cure of their diseases, from any part of the Province, without partiality or preference." This seems to me eminently wise, since it takes from contributors, Managers, and treasurer, the temptation to use for any purpose, it matters not how wise and provident such purpose might appear at the time, the capital fund of the institution.

One feature in the history of the Hospital, connected with this subject, I think is deserving of notice, and this is that the present excellent treasurer, Mr. John T. Lewis, who has served the institution now for 34 years, was preceded by his father, uncle, and grandfather, three generations of the same family, whose united term of service counts to but four years less than a century. We Americans are prone to regard with envy the stable habits of our mother country, and to fancy that America rarely exhibits families, as is so often seen in England, in which successive generations show the solid advantages of inherited integrity and fitness for public office. In this Hospital, we have at least one instance of the descent of virtue and charity from grandfather to grandson.

After ascribing all honor to the Managers for their admirable control of the institution, it is right and proper that I should refer to the medical and surgical staff of the city department. Between the years 1853 and 1876, there have been admitted into the city department 41,379 patients, the whole medical and surgical care and responsibility of which cases rest with the staff. Many of these cases belong to the recent accident class, those dreadful injuries of all and every possible kind, from sprains or simple fractures, up to the most disastrous railroad accidents, explosions in fire-arms or cartridge factories, burns and scalds, indeed, the whole miserable black catalogue of injuries to which the human frame is exposed. Other cases are those of the deadly fevers, typhoid, remitting, and intermittent, dysenteries, the various local inflammations, the consumptions, catarrhs, cancers, and all the sad list of medical woes which make hospitals so necessary. I cite these particular names of things so unpalatable, in order that the lay reader may, perhaps, catch some faint idea of what the work of the medical and surgical staff is in this Hospital. The whole of this dreary toil amidst the sick and wounded, the great central object of the Hospital, is done by the staff, as is the work of the Managers, without money emolument. It has been performed now by the medical men of Philadelphia for one hundred and twenty-five years, as one of the many charitable works of the profession. Until the year 1871, a small fee, ten dollars, was charged for admission to the clinical lectures, the proceeds of which were applied, at the request of the staff, to build up the very handsome medical library of the Hospital, to which I have already referred. But, in the year just mentioned, the staff proposed to the Board that they should abandon even this small fee.

and make the lectures entirely free of expense to all students of respectable colleges. This was done. So let it be put on record in the history of the Hospital, that the daily visiting and care of the sick and wounded in the city Hospital, is most faithfully performed, in all its length and breadth, gratuitously, by the medical and surgical staff.

I take great pride as a citizen of Philadelphia and of this State in the history of this oldest Hospital in the State, since it shows forth the admirable manner in which its interests have been served, and its funds husbanded and increased by the gentlemen who have served it. Let us not fail to do justice to the men who have managed this Hospital so well. Hear what a Chief Justice said in 1834, about a case which came before the court, of a devise establishing an Orphan House, for the maintenance and education of poor orphan children. The trust had been abused and the Chief Justice said it was "an additional instance of the futility of private charities," and that "even when established by law, and provided with the conservative apparatus of visitation, inspection, and whatever ingenuity could contrive, these misdirected efforts of benevolence had conduced but to the emoluments of the agents intrusted with their care. So it would ever be, when the vision of the visitor was not sharpened by individual interest." The case is given by Mr. Binney in his argument in the Girard case. In a foot-note to the case Mr. Binney says: "This is a melancholy picture of charitable gifts and institutions; but, while its resemblance to individual cases may be admitted—for what institutions are not sometimes abused?—we should, for the honor of humanity, be slow to admit its accuracy in point of general resemblance. We must all know many charities which have been faithfully, disinterestedly, and most beneficially administered. The city of Philadelphia has many of them, and, it is to be hoped, ever will have them, and as in times past they have been, so we may predict that in all future time they will continue to be, as much a source of praise to the giver, of honor to the visitors and trustees, as they have been and will be of comfort, relief, and improvement to their manifold objects." I cannot doubt that, in writing these words, Mr. Binney may have thought of this very Hospital, for often have I heard him speak with great satisfaction and commendation of its management.

I have now brought the history of this institution, during the past twenty-five years, to a conclusion, and I might end my labor here, but, in studying the past of anything that has a continuous existence, the mind travels inevitably into the future, and I feel that my work would be unfinished, were I to say nothing as to the probable future of the Hospital.

Two points in particular press upon my thoughts in considering the future of the Hospital—one is the direction in which its progressive development ought to take place—and the other is the fact which should be known to all men, who feel an interest in its success, that it needs a large addition to its funds, if it is to go on increasing in usefulness as it has done in the past.

The Hospital was chartered for the "reception and relief of lunatics, and other distempered and sick poor within this Province," as the charter recites in one paragraph, or for "the entertainment and cure of the sick and distempered poor," as the words run in another paragraph. It is fair to presume that its duty is to distribute its care in due proportion to these different classes of the sick. The dew of its charity should fall upon all classes of the sick and wounded poor, in as fair a proportion as it is possible for the Hospital to arrange and provide for. It is for the Managers to decide how to expend the funds given or bequeathed to the Hospital so as best to realize this end.

I can think of no better guide for the Hospital authorities in this matter, than the determination by reliable vital statistics, of the proportion of deaths in a large community, caused by the three great divisions of disease, received into this Hospital—medical, surgical, and insane. This will give a standard to decide the direction in which a hospital, created and maintained by the gifts and legacies of the charitable, ought to seek to develop itself.

To obtain this standard, I shall take first the Report of the Registrar General of England, the best, probably, the world affords, and ascertain the proportion of deaths from medical and surgical causes in all England, and then in the city of London. In this way, we shall find the relative proportion of deaths from these two chief groups of causes, first, in the rural and town populations together, and then in the largest city in the world. I shall then do the same thing for our own city of Philadelphia. I have taken the year 1857 for England, as this is the last report I have been able to find, and the year 1874 for this city.

In 1857, the whole number of deaths in all England was 419,815. Of this total, the deaths from surgical diseases were 32,157. I include amongst these the deaths from syphilis, hemorrhage, abscess, ulcer, fistula, mortification, cancer, scrofula, aneurism, hernia, ileus, intussusception, stricture of the intestinal canal, stone, cystitis, stricture of the urethra, ovarian dropsy, carbuncle, diseases of the joints, phlegmon, spina bifida and other malformations, poison, burns and scalds, hanging and suffocation, drowning, fractures and contusions, wounds, and other violence. Of these causes of death, not a few would come into the hands of the physician, whether in private or hospital practice; as some of the syphilitic cases, of those from hemorrhage, from cancer, scrofula, ileus, intussusception, stricture of the urethra, cystitis, and poison; but I have preferred to consider them all surgical, in order to make sure that the result, which, at first view, is surprising, should not by any chance be incorrect.

I find that of the whole number of deaths in all England, 419,815, the number from surgical causes was 32,157, or 7.65 per cent. In London, the whole number of deaths was 59,103, of which those from surgical causes were 4934, or 8.34 per cent., showing that a larger proportion, as might have been expected, occurs in a large city, than in the general population of a whole country.

In this city, in the year 1874, the whole number of deaths was 16,254. The number of deaths from the surgical causes enumerated above was 992, or 6.1 per cent.

In 1857, the deaths from insanity in all England, as given in the Registrar General's Report, were only 403. This, of course, does not give the real number of deaths of insane persons. But I find, in Bucknill and Tuke's Psychological Medicine, p. 298, the following statement as to the mortality of the insane: "From the Lunacy Report of the present year (1861), we learn the annual rate of mortality during five years ending December 31, 1858. The deaths (calculated on the mean number resident, over 20,225) amounted to 10.97 per cent." This proportion would give 2218 per annum, and, assuming that the same number died in 1857 as in 1861, we should have a percentage of 55 hundredths of one per cent.

In this city, of the whole number of deaths in 1874, given in the Report of the Board of Health to the Mayor, 16,254, only three are to be found under the head of insanity. The insane department of this Hospital, alone, reports for that year 46 deaths. But, as we have, probably, a much safer ratio in the English Reports, I shall not attempt to give that for our city.

The deaths in all England, in 1857, from obstetrical causes, including the deaths in childbirth, and those from puerperal fever, were 2787, or a percentage of 66 hundredths of one per cent. of the whole number of deaths.

These facts show that something more than 91 per cent. of all the deaths in England in 1857 were caused by the varieties of disease usually denominated medical, and that a hospital which is to take equal care of all classes of the sick and wounded, must expend over 90 per cent. of its charitable endowment on the medical wards. These proportions seem, at first view, incredible, and yet, if the above calculations are correct, the results must be as they are here set down. And, when we reflect how numerous are the cases of consumption, of typhoid and typhus fever, scarlet fever, pneumonia, pleurisy, rheumatism, catarrh, dysentery, diarrhœa, remittent and intermittent fevers, we need not be so much surprised. Even in the most deadly wars, it is not the loss of life in battle or from wounds that weakens armies; it is the train of diseases that break out in camp, in forced marches or retreats, or in sieges, which cause much the greater part of the whole mortality.

To render these observations of use as a guide in the future development of a hospital like this one, it would be necessary to eliminate from the whole number of deaths from medical causes, all such as are not received in this hospital—still-births, many of the diseases of children, and contagious diseases in general—but, as my object is rather to suggest what may be necessary in the future, than what is exactly appropriate at the present time, I shall pursue the matter no further. More precise and particular calculations can be made whenever it may become proper to do so.

It is well known to all who are familiar with the history of the Pennsylvania Hospital, that it has long been pre-eminently a surgical hospital. Thus, in the five years 1852–56 inclusive, the whole number of admissions was 9556, of which 5717 were surgical and 3839 medical, or 59.82 per cent. surgical. In the five years 1872–76 the whole number of cases was 10,057, of which 6416 were surgical and 3641 medical, or 63.79 per cent. surgical. So that the hospital has been in the habit of devoting considerably more than half of its funds to the care of surgical cases occurring in the city or in its environs, though, out of the whole number of deaths in a community, as I have explained, not more than $7\frac{1}{2}$ to $8\frac{1}{2}$ per cent. are due to surgical diseases. This great disparity in the proportion of the surgical to medical cases, has been the result of a custom of this hospital, already referred to several times, of receiving all recent accidents, brought to its doors within twenty-four hours of their occurrence, without question. This custom was doubtless the fruit of a charitable necessity. For many years there was no proper hospital accommodation in the city, for surgical cases, except in this institution, and it became one of the fixed habits of the poor to carry their diseased friends and relatives to this one sure refuge. Not only so, but the easy classes of society, and the great manufacturing establishments, knowing this rule of the hospital, to take all recent accidents without question, naturally aided in establishing this almost universal custom. So predominant was the importance of the surgical wards that in 1866, when, as I have related before, there was some doubt as to whether some of the wards would not have to be closed, the only ones hinted at or mentioned, were the medical. This miserable necessity was, however, avoided, happily for the reputation of the hospital.

Within a few years the Blockley Hospital has been taking a much larger number of recent accidents than in previous times. The city now supplies that hospital with an ambulance, which being sent for from the police stations when accidents occur, carries patients to its wards from all parts of the city.[1] Other hospitals have been erected—the Episcopal, the Presbyterian, the University, and, at this very time, the Jefferson Medical College is building one to be connected with its school. These increased accommodations for the sick and wounded cannot fail to lessen the demands to be made upon the Pennsylvania Hospital, and it is reasonable to suppose that the pressure upon this latter for surgical patients will diminish. As the whole number of surgical cases in the community is so much less than the medical, and as all the new foundations will soon be ready to take their proportion of accidents, we may safely assume that the time has now come, or is at hand, when this charity may prepare to expand the accommodations for medical cases, in a larger proportion than it has yet been able to do.

As to the Insane Department of this Hospital, it

[1] The Managers of the Pennsylvania Hospital have recently decided to have an ambulance attached to this Hospital.

is already so large in proportion to that for the sick and wounded, that it will scarcely need any further expansion for many years to come. And, if we bear in mind the fact that, in all England, the proportion of deaths from insanity to the whole number, was but fifty-five hundredths of one per cent., it does certainly seem, that this foundation is doing as much for the insane at the present time, as its endowment makes proper and necessary.

One thing more I may say in regard to the surgical department of the hospital. It has already been stated that the Blockley Hospital maintains an ambulance of its own. The University Hospital also maintains one. These ambulances are sent for from the police stations to the scene of a recent accident and, of course, convey the sufferers to the hospitals to which they are attached, often carrying the injured persons considerable distances, and past the doors of this and other hospitals. It has been suggested, and I think with good reason, that the municipal authorities of the city be invited to establish city ambulances, perhaps in connection with the fire department, which might be sent for when accidents occur, with directions to carry the patients to the nearest hospital prepared for their reception. This system would have two great advantages. It would lessen, in many cases, the distances over which the sufferers have to be transported, and it would diminish the heavy taxation borne by the city, for the support of the Blockley Hospital, by diverting from its wards many surgical cases that would then be received into, and supported by, the private charitable institutions ready and willing to take care of them.

The other point connected with the future career of this Hospital, to which I desired to call attention, was its need for a larger endowment. It requires more funds in order to continue what it has been doing for several years past, in a more complete and effective manner, or to increase, as it ought to be enabled to do, the number of sick to be received within its walls.

The expenses have been increasing from two principal causes—the diminution in the number of pay-patients in proportion to the free, and the great increase in the cost of living. In 1856, twenty years since, the whole number of patients admitted was 1714, of which number 1154 were poor and 560 pay. The expenses were $34,657.83, of which amount $9,185.47 were received from the board of patients. In 1876 the admissions were 1638, of which 1270 were poor and 368 pay. The expenses were $62,666.22, of which sum $9,766.80 were received for board, so that it cost the Hospital $28,028.39 more to support, in 1876, a number of patients less by 76 than in 1856, yet the amount received for board was very nearly the same.

Though the whole number of patients in 1876 was less than in 1856, it is probable that this diminution was owing to some temporary cause, for I find, on comparing periods of five years, that there has been a very decided increase. In the five years 1851 to 1856 the whole number was 8,845, while in the five years, 1872 to 1876, it was 9,250, a difference in the five years of 405.

It is clear, therefore, that the funds of the Hospital, for the maintenance of the department for the sick and wounded, ought to be increased as soon as possible, and in a very considerable degree.

The other branch of the Hospital, the Insane Department, also needs additional endowment. This department has had most remarkable success. As stated before, it has received, of the income from the vested capital in the last thirty years, $159,996.36, or but $4,571.32 per annum. And yet its expenditures are very heavy. I find that, for the last five years, its annual expenditure has varied from $172,000 to $214,000. These large sums were paid almost wholly by the board received from the paying patients. Indeed, in the last year, 1875, it appears to have been more than self-supporting, since the total expenditures were $201,366.53, and the net receipts $205,532.70.

This branch supports, on these means, a good many poor patients who pay nothing, and a number of others who are received at a rate of board so moderate, that it does not pay the cost of their support. During the last five years, the number of free patients has varied from 35 in 1873, to 43 in 1871 and 1872, and 51 in 1875. Since its opening in 1841, it has received 7167 patients in all, of which number 1532 were taken without charge, and about as many more paid less than the cost of their support.

So that this department is now, and has been, doing

all that it can afford to do for the poor. To extend its care to a yet larger number, it must have an increase of its funds. In the last report, that of 1875, it is stated that, "The claimants for admission on the part of those unable to pay the full cost of their support, are constantly increasing, and are far beyond the resources of the Institution. Many of them are of the greatest interest and curable. It is to meet these applications, and to provide everything that will promote additional comforts, greater happiness, and give better chances of restoration for all its patients, that the Institution needs large additions to its resources, and especially a great increase of the permanent fund, which has been liberally started by a few benevolent individuals.

When free beds are established, they are for indigent, recent, and supposed curable cases only; and, judging by past experience, when thus used, every such bed may be expected to be the means of restoring to reason and to society, from one to two patients in every year the Hospital shall exist."

To all who have read this history of the last twenty-five years of the Pennsylvania Hospital, it must be plain that, for the extensive good it has done and is still doing, it is not the wealthy institution which many suppose it to be. I think I have shown, on the contrary, that it has been compelled to exceed constantly its income, and that it has never been able to attain to that degree of usefulness, in its city department especially, which it might reach had it more abundant means. The history has exhibited the

Managers embarrassed, hampered, distressed, at times despondent, obliged to go before the public, hat in hand, so to speak, to implore the gift of funds to make up its annual deficiencies. What toil, what stripes, what rebuffs, have they not been forced to endure? The hospital may be likened to that noblest sight in the world, the good man struggling with adversity.

I have portrayed, too, the spotless integrity, the steady and devoted loyalty to the right, the reputation undimmed even by a suspicion, with which its affairs have been administered. Having shown this noble picture of what has been accomplished by this charity, shall I hesitate to advise any one who desires to see the gracious fruit of his liberality while he yet lives, or who may wish to leave a lasting good behind him, not to forget that here is an institution, one of the antiquities of our young country, the history of which shows forth only the finest uses of charity?

I will venture to add that, to me personally, it appears most wise to give money to the general endowment fund, in order that the Board of Managers, that active, intelligent body which never dies, never wastes, never misappropriates, may apply the income of the capital in such manner for the general good of all the poor, as time and progress shall declare to be most wise and necessary.

If any one should wish to perpetuate the name of some beloved relative, or to illustrate his own name and family, let him endow one or more free beds to be called after the person for whom they are endowed. I doubt even whether it is wise to choose between the two departments. Who can know, at this moment of time, what may be the necessities of a great hospital in the future? To the Managers, it appears to me, it would be best to leave the appropriation of the income in such direction in the distant future as time and the growth of society shall show to be necessary.

And now at length I come to the end of my labor. The task I have essayed, and am about to conclude, has been a labor of love. I am, and have always been, a citizen of Philadelphia. I was brought up in a medical family, and imbibed from my father, who served the hospital faithfully for ten years, a sentiment towards this institution which touched upon the romantic. And he and I were by no means singular in this, for it is a fact, and I wish to put this on record, that there always has been amongst our citizens a peculiar sentiment of tenderness, mingled with the pride felt for the Pennsylvania Hospital. This sentiment was composed largely of love, untouched by any fear of abuse. Such has been the management throughout its career that no one suspected, or dreaded, anything like misapplication of its funds. Perfect love had, indeed, cast out fear in this one, at least, of our public institutions. The hospital is now, and ever has been, one of the embellishments of Philadelphia. In this city, for now so many years, its large square of ground, open to the air and light, except for its neat and simple, but striking mass of buildings, and its noble girdle of trees, which has so long surrounded the square, has had, I cannot but fancy, something to do with the interest felt by the citizens in the institution. The circlet of superb foliage which marked, like a crown, the house of the poor sick, was visible from all parts of the city, and could not be seen by those who knew what it marked, and who had any sense of the beauty and fitness of things, without raising in the mind a sense of gratitude, that there the sick and wounded who were homeless, might find a refuge, and one of pride that the city could boast so great an embellishment.

# APPENDIX.

## I.

## MANAGERS AND TREASURERS.

*The following is a list of those who have served as Managers and Treasurers from the commencement of the Institution to the present time; with the date of their respective elections, and the length of time they continued in office.*

| Managers. | Elected. | Resigned. | Served the Institution. |
|---|---|---|---|
| Joshua Crosby | 1751 | 1755 | 4 years (died). |
| Benjamin Franklin | 1751 | 1757 | 6 years. |
| Thomas Bond | 1751 | 1752 | 1 year. |
| Samuel Hazard | 1751 | 1754 | 3 years. |
| Richard Peters | 1751 | 1752 | 1 year. |
| Israel Pemberton, Jr. | 1751 | 1779 | 28 years. |
| Samuel Rhoads | 1751 | 1781 | 30 years. |
| Hugh Roberts | 1751 | 1756 | 5 years. |
| Joseph Morris | 1751 | 1757 | 6 years. |
| John Smith | 1751, 1761 | 1756, 1762 | 6 years. |
| Evan Morgan | 1751, 1753 | 1752, 1763 | 11 years. |
| Charles Norris | 1751 | 1752 | 1 year. |
| Isaac Jones | 1752, 1760, 1764 | 1756, 1762, 1773 | 15 years and 5 months (died). |
| John Reynell | 1752 | 1780 | 28 years. |
| William Griffitts | 1752 | 1753 | 1 year and 5 months. |
| Thomas Lawrence, Jr. | 1752 | 1753 | 1 year. |
| Joseph Fox | 1753 | 1756 | 2 years and 7 months. |
| William Grant | 1754 | 1756 | 2 years. |
| Thomas Crosby | 1755 | 1757 | 1 year and 11 months. |
| Daniel Roberdeau | 1756, 1766 | 1758, 1776 | 12 years. |
| Charles Jones | 1756 | 1761 | 5 years. |
| Isaac Greenleaf | 1756 | 1771 | 15 years.  [(died). |
| Joseph Richardson, Mer't | 1756 | 1770 | 17 years and 6 months |
| Jacob Duchee | 1756 | 1758 | 1 year and 9 months. |
| Plunket Fleeson | 1757 | 1759 | 2 years. |
| Anthony Benezet | 1757 | 1758 | 1 year. |
| John Sayre | 1757 | 1758 | 9 months. |
| Stephen Shewell | 1758 | 1760 | 2 years. |
| Thomas Gordon | 1758 | 1766 | 8 years. |

| Managers. | Elected. | Resigned | Served the Institution. |
|---|---|---|---|
| Samuel Mifflin | 1758 | 1760 | 2 years. |
| James Pemberton | 1758 | 1780 | 22 years. |
| Jacob Lewis | 1759 | 1774 | 15 years.    [(died). |
| John Mease | 1760 | 1768 | 7 years and 10 months |
| Henry Harrison | 1762 | 1766 | 3 y'rs and 9 mo's (died). |
| Thomas Wharton | 1762 | 1769 | 7 years. |
| John Gibson | {1763<br>{1767 | 1764}<br>1770} | 3 years and 7 months. |
| Joseph Redmon | 1766 | 1767 | 1 year and 1 month. |
| John Nixon | 1768 | 1772 | 4 years. |
| Joseph Morris | 1769 | 1781 | 12 years. |
| *Isaac Cox | 1770 | 1776 | 5 y'rs and 8 mo's (died). |
| William Logan | 1770 | 1775 | 4 years and 6 months. |
| Thomas Mifflin | 1771 | 1773 | 1 year and 11 months. |
| Thomas Wharton | 1772 | 1779 | 7 years. |
| Edward Penington | 1773 | 1779 | 6 years. |
| Robert Strettell Jones | 1773 | 1781 | 8 years. |
| George Roberts | 1774 | 1776 | 2 years and 3 months. |
| Thomas Fisher | 1775 | 1776 | 1 year and 3 months. |
| Joseph Swift | 1776 | 1786 | 9 years and 9 months. |
| William West | 1776 | 1778 | 2 years. |
| Jacob Shoemaker | 1776 | 1781 | 5 years. |
| William Morrell | 1776 | 1782 | 6 years and 8 months. |
| Samuel Powell | 1778 | 1780 | 2 years. |
| Joshua Howell | 1779 | 1782 | 3 years. |
| Samuel Pleasants | 1779 | 1781 | 2 years. |
| Peter Reeve | 1779 | 1786 | 7 years. |
| George Mifflin | 1780 | 1785 | 5 y'rs and 2 mo's (died). |
| Thomas Franklin | 1780 | 1783 | 3 years. |
| Tench Coxe | 1780 | 1781 | 1 year. |
| Reynold Keene | 1781 | 1790 | 9 years and 7 months. |
| Jonathan Shoemaker | 1781 | 1790 | 9 years and 1 month. |
| Owen Jones, Jr. | 1781 | 1795 | 13 years and 9 months. |
| Isaac Wharton | 1781 | 1784 | 3 years. |
| Josiah Hewes | 1781 | 1812 | 30 years and 5 months. |
| John Morton | 1781 | 1785 | 3 years and 8 months. |
| Adam Hubley | 1782 | 1784 | 2 years and 4 months. |
| Nathaniel Falconer | {1782<br>{1784 | 1783}<br>1790} | 6 years and 6 months. |
| Andrew Doz | 1783 | 1788 | 5 years. |
| Thomas Moore | 1783 | 1788 | 5 years. |
| Samuel Howell | 1784 | 1789 | 4 years and 5 months. |
| William Hall | 1785 | 1787 | 1 year and 11 months. |
| Samuel Coates | 1785 | 1825 | 40 years and 4 months. |
| John Paschall | 1786 | 1795 | 8 years and 10 months |
| Thomas Penrose | 1786 | 1798 | 12 years.    [(died). |

\* It appears from the minutes of the Board, that Isaac Cox was lost at sea, on his return from the Island of New Providence, in the winter of 1775-6.

| Managers. | Elected. | Resigned. | Served the Institution. |
|---|---|---|---|
| Richard Rundle | 1787 | 1789 | 2 years. |
| Samuel Clark | 1788 | 1802 | 13 years and 6 months |
| Pattison Hartshorne | 1788 | 1823 | 35 years.    [(died). |
| Elliston Perot | 1789 | 1806 | 17 years and 2 months. |
| Bartholomew Wistar | 1789 | 1796 | 7 years. |
| Cornelius Barnes | 1790 | 1793 | 3 y'rs and 5 mo's (died). |
| Lawrence Seckel | 1790 | 1820 | 29 years and 9 months. |
| William McMurtrie | 1791 | 1794 | 3 years.    [(died). |
| Thomas Morris | 1793 | 1809 | 15 years and 11 months |
| Samuel M. Fox | 1794 | 1797 | 3 years. |
| Robert Waln | 1795 | 1800 | 5 years and 2 months. |
| James Smith, Jr. | 1795 | 1805 | 10 years. |
| Israel Pleasants | 1796 | 1800 | 4 years. |
| John Dorsey | 1797 | 1804 | 7 years. |
| Robert Smith, Merchant | 1798 | 1805 | 7 years. |
| Zaccheus Collins | 1800 | 1822 | 22 years. |
| Paschall Hollingsworth | 1800 | 1812 | 12 years. |
| Richard Wistar | 1803 | 1806 | 3 years and 4 months. |
| Joseph Lownes | 1804 | 1820 | 16 years. |
| Peter Brown | 1805 | 1811 | 6 y'rs and 7 mo's (died). |
| Edward Penington | 1805 | 1820 | 15 years. |
| Zachariah Poulson | 1806 | 1808 | 1 year and 10 months. |
| William Poyntell | 1806 | 1811 | 5 y'rs and 2 mo's (died). |
| Thomas Stewardson | 1808 | 1841 | 33 years and 2 months |
| Thomas P. Cope | 1809 | 1828 | 19 years.    [(died). |
| Reeve Lewis | 1811 | 1814 | 3 years and 3 months. |
| Joseph S. Morris | 1811 | 1817 | 5 y'rs and 3 mo's (died). |
| Samuel W. Fisher | 1812 | 1817 | 4 y'rs and 9 mo's (died). |
| Joseph Watson | 1812 | 1824 | 12 years and 5 months. |
| Mordecai Lewis | {1814<br>{1828 | 1818}<br>1849} | 24 years and 9 months. |
| Israel Cope | 1817 | 1828 | 11 years. |
| Thomas Morris | 1817 | 1840 | 23 years and 9 months. |
| Henry Hollingsworth | 1818 | 1823 | 5 years and 6 months. |
| Alexander Elmslie | 1820 | 1827 | 7 years. |
| Matthew L. Bevan | 1820 | 1828 | 7 years and 10 months. |
| Joseph Johnson | 1820 | 1828 | 7 years and 10 months. |
| William L. Hodge | 1822 | 1824 | 2 years. |
| Roberts Vaux | 1823 | 1834 | 11 years. |
| Charles Roberts | 1823 | 1844 | 21 years and 3 months. |
| William W. Fisher | 1824 | 1838 | 13 y's and 8 mo's (died). |
| Charles Watson | 1824 | 1846 | 21 years and 2 months. |
| John Paul | 1825 | 1844 | 18 y's and 8 mo's (died). |
| Joseph R. Jenks | 1827 | 1828 | 10 months. |
| Joseph Price | 1828 | 1845 | 17 years and 6 months. |
| Alexander W. Johnson | 1828 | 1848 | 20 years and 8 months. |
| John J. Smith | 1828 | 1836 | 8 years and 7 months. |

| Managers. | Elected. | Resigned. | Served the Institution. |
|---|---|---|---|
| Bartholomew Wistar | 1828 | 1841 | 13 y's and 5 mo's (died). |
| Lawrence Lewis | 1834 | 1855 | 21 y's and 7 mo's (died). |
| James R. Greeves | (1836<br>(1842 | 1838)<br>1866) | 25 years. |
| George Roberts Smith | 1838 | 1850 | 12 years and 4 months. |
| Nathan Dunn | 1838 | 1842 | 4 years. |
| William B. Fling | 1841 | 1856 | 15 years. |
| Frederick Brown | 1841 | 1864 | 22 y's and 7 mo's (d'd). |
| Isaac Elliott | 1841 | 1842 | 1 year and 2 months. |
| George Stewardson | 1842 | 1855 | 13 years and 4 months. |
| Jacob G. Morris | 1844 | 1854 | 10 years (died). |
| Mordecai L. Dawson | 1844 | 1872 | 27 y's and 11 mo's (d'd). |
| Clement C. Biddle | 1846 | 1855 | 9 y's and 6 mo's (died). |
| John Farnum | 1846 | 1872 | 26 y's and 4 mo's (d'd). |
| Mordecai D. Lewis | 1848 | 1861 | 12 y's and 1 mo. (died). |
| William Biddle | 1849 | | |
| John M. Whitall | 1851 | 1867 | 16 years and 3 months. |
| Alexander J. Derbyshire | 1855 | | |
| Samuel Mason | 1855 | | |
| S. Morris Waln | 1855 | 1870 | 15 y's and 3 mo's (d'd). |
| Samuel Welsh | 1856 | | |
| Joseph S. Lewis | 1856 | 1857 | 1 year and 8 months. |
| Wistar Morris | 1857 | | |
| Caleb Cope | 1861 | 1868 | 7 years and 5 months. |
| Adolph E. Borie | 1864 | 1868 | 4 years and 3 months. |
| Jacob P. Jones | 1866 | | |
| Benjamin H. Shoemaker | 1867 | | |
| Alexander Biddle | 1868 | | |
| Edward Y. Townsend | 1868 | 1869 | 5 months. |
| Joseph B. Townsend | 1869 | | |
| Joseph C. Turnpenny | 1870 | | |
| John J. Thompson | 1872 | 1875 | 2 y's and 11 mo's (died). |
| T. Wistar Brown | 1872 | | |
| Henry Haines | 1875 | | |

Of the above, the following were the successive Presidents of the Board:—

| | Years. | | Years. |
|---|---|---|---|
| 1. Joshua Crosby | 4 | 9. Samuel Coates | 13 |
| 2. Benjamin Franklin | 2 | 10. Thomas Stewardson | 16 |
| 3. John Reynell | 23 | 11. John Paul | 3 |
| 4. Samuel Rhoads | 1 | 12. Mordecai Lewis | 5 |
| 5. Peter Reeve | 5 | 13. Lawrence Lewis | $6\frac{1}{2}$ |
| 6. Samuel Howell | 3 | 14. Mordecai L. Dawson | $16\frac{3}{4}$ |
| 7. Reynold Keen | 1 | 15. William Biddle | |
| 8. Josiah Hewes | 22 | | |

| Treasurers. | Elected. | Resigned. | Served the Institution. |
|---|---|---|---|
| John Reynell | 1751 | 1752 | 1 year. |
| Charles Norris | 1752 | 1756 | 4 years. |
| Hugh Roberts | 1756 | 1768 | 12 years. |
| Samuel P. Moore | 1768 | 1769 | 1 year. |
| Thomas Wharton | 1769 | 1772 | 3 years. |
| Joseph King | 1772 | 1773 | 13 months (died). |
| Joseph Hilborn | 1773 | 1780 | 7 years. |
| Mordecai Lewis | 1780 | 1799 | 18 y's and 8 mo's (died). |
| Joseph S. Lewis | 1799 | 1826 | 27 years. |
| Samuel N. Lewis | 1826 | 1841 | 14 y's and 2 mo's (died). |
| John T. Lewis | 1841 | | |

## 11.

## MEDICAL OFFICERS.

*The following are the names of the gentlemen who have served the Institution as Physicians and Surgeons, in the order of their appointment; together with the date of their resignation or death, and their respective periods of service.*

| Physicians and Surgeons. | Elected. | Resigned. | Served the Institution. |
|---|---|---|---|
| Lloyd Zachary | 1751 | 1753 | 1 year and 5 months. |
| Thomas Bond | 1751 | 1784 | 32 years and 6 months |
| Phineas Bond | 1751 | 1773 | 21 y's and 8 mo's (died). |
| Thomas Cadwalader | 1751 | 1777 | 25 years and 6 months. |
| Samuel Preston Moore | 1751 | 1759 | 7 years and 6 months. |
| John Redman | 1751 | 1780 | 28 years and 6 months. |
| William Shippen | 1753 | 1778 | 25 years and 2 months. |
| Cadwalader Evans | 1759 | 1773 | 14 y's and 1 mo. (died). |
| John Morgan | 1773 / 1778 | 1777 / 1783 | 8 years and 11 months. |
| Charles Moore | 1773 | 1774 | 10 months. |
| Adam Kuhn | 1774 / 1782 | 1781 / 1798 | 22 years and 6 months. |
| Thomas Parke | 1777 | 1823 | 45 years and 9 months. |
| James Hutchinson | 1777 / 1779 | 1778 / 1793 | 15 years (died). |
| William Shippen, Jr. | 1778 / 1791 | 1779 / 1802 | 11 y'rs and 11 months. |
| John Jones | 1780 | 1791 | 11 y's and 1 mo. (died). |
| Benjamin Rush | 1783 | 1813 | 29 years and 10 months |
| John Foulke | 1784 | 1794 | 10 years.   [(died). |
| Caspar Wistar | 1793 | 1810 | 16 years and 5 months. |
| Philip Syng Physick | 1794 | 1816 | 22 years and 1 month. |
| Benjamin Smith Barton | 1798 | 1815 | 17 years and 10 months. |
| John Redman Coxe | 1802 | 1807 | 4 years and 9 months. |
| Thomas C. James | 1807 | 1832 | 25 y'rs and 10 months. |
| John Syng Dorsey | 1810 | 1818 | 8 y'rs and 6 mo's (died). |
| Joseph Hartshorne | 1810 | 1821 | 11 years and 2 months. |
| John C. Otto | 1813 | 1835 | 22 years and 4 months. |
| Samuel Colhoun | 1816 | 1821 | 5 years. |
| Joseph Parrish | 1816 | 1829 | 12 years and 8 months. |

| Physicians and Surgeons. | Elected. | Resigned | Served the Institution. |
| --- | --- | --- | --- |
| Thomas T. Hewson | 1818 | 1835 | 16 years and 5 months. |
| John Moore | 1820 | 1829 | 9 years. |
| William Price | 1821 | 1823 | 1 year and 10 months. |
| John Wilson Moore | 1821 | 1827 | 5 years and 3 months. |
| Samuel Emlen | 1823 | 1828 | 5 years (died). |
| John Rhea Barton | 1823 | 1836 | 13 years and 5 months. |
| John K. Mitchell | 1827 | 1834 | 7 years. |
| Benjamin H. Coates | 1828 | 1841 | 12 years and 9 months. |
| Thomas Harris | 1829 | 1840 | 11 years and 9 months. |
| Charles Lukens | 1829 | 1839 | 10 years and 3 months. |
| Hugh L. Hodge | 1832 | 1854 | 21 years and 3 months. |
| William Rush | 1834 | 1837 | 3 years and 5 months. |
| George B. Wood | 1835 | 1859 | 23 years and 6 months. |
| Jacob Randolph | 1835 | 1848 | 12 y's and 10 mo's (d'd). |
| George W. Norris | 1836 | 1863 | 27 years. |
| Thomas Stewardson | 1838 | 1845 | 7 years. |
| Charles D. Meigs | 1838 | 1849 | 10 y'rs and 10 months. |
| Edward Peace | 1840 | 1861 | 20 years and 1 month. |
| William Pepper | 1842 | 1858 | 16 years and 7 months. |
| William W. Gerhard | 1845 | 1868 | 23 years. |
| George Fox | 1848 | 1854 | 6 years. |
| Joseph Carson | 1849 | 1854 | 4 years and 10 months. |
| John Neill | 1852 | 1859 | 7 years and 1 month. |
| Joseph Pancoast | 1854 | 1864 | 9 years and 11 months. |
| James J. Levick | 1856 | 1868 | 12 years and 5 months. |
| John Forsythe Meigs | 1859 | | |
| Edward Hartshorne | 1859 | 1865 | 5 years and 9 months. |
| Francis Gurney Smith | 1859 | 1864 | 5 years and 7 months. |
| Addinell Hewson | 1861 | | |
| William Hunt | 1863 | | |
| Thomas Geo. Morton | 1863 | | |
| Jacob M. DaCosta | 1865 | | |
| D. Hayes Agnew | 1865 | 1871 | 6 years and 2 months. |
| James H. Hutchinson | 1868 | | |
| J. Aitken Meigs | 1868 | | |
| Richard J. Levis | 1871 | | |

## MEDICAL APPRENTICES AND RESIDENT PHYSICIANS.

*The Apprentices were Students of Medicine when indentured to the Hospital, and usually graduated before leaving it.*

|  | From. | To. | Served. |
|---|---|---|---|
| Jacob Ehrenzeller | 1773 | 1778 | 5 years. |
| William Gardner | 1786 | 1791 | 5 years. |
| Edward Cutbush | 1790 | 1794 | 4 years. |
| Samuel Cooper | 1792 | 1797 | 5 years. |
| Thomas Horsefield | 1794 | 1799 | 5 years. |
| George Lee | 1798 | 1802 | 4 years (died). |
| James Hutchinson, Jr. | 1799 | 1804 | 5 years. |
| Joseph Hartshorne | 1801 | 1806 | 5 years. |
| Samuel C. Hopkins | 1804 | 1808 | 4 years. |
| Thomas Bryant, M.D. | 1806 | 1807 | 1 year. |
| Philip Thornton | 1806 | 1808 | 1 year and 9 months. |
| Samuel Betton, M.D. | 1808 | 1808 | 6 months. |
| John Wilson Moore | 1808 | 1813 | 5 years. |
| Benjamin S. Janney | 1808 | 1813 | 5 years. |
| Wm. P. C. Barton, M.D. | 1809 | 1809 | 4 months. |
| Samuel Colhoun, M.D. | 1809 | 1810 | 1 year. |
| Theodore Benson | 1810 | 1813 | 3 years (died). |
| John Rhea Barton | 1813 | 1818 | 5 years. |
| William Price, M.D. | 1813 | 1814 | 1 year. |
| Benjamin H. Coates | 1814 | 1819 | 5 years. |
| Jason O'B. Lawrence, M.D. | 1814 | 1815 | 6 months. |
| Warwick P. Miller | 1815 | 1819 | 4 years (died). |
| George Balfour | 1818 | 1819 | 9 months. |
| Thomas H. Ritchie | 1819 | 1823 | 4 years. |
| Reynell Coates | 1819 | 1823 | 4 years. |
| Thomas Flanner | 1819 | 1820 | 9 months. |
| Robert J. Clark, M.D. | 1820 | 1821 | 9 months. |
| Southey H. Satchell, M.D. | 1823 | 1824 | 1 year. |
| Charles B. Jaudon, M.D. | 1823 | 1824 | 10 months. |

The three last-named gentlemen served for unfinished terms of preceding apprentices. From this time, it was resolved to elect graduates of medicine only as

## RESIDENT PHYSICIANS.

| | From. | To. | Served. |
|---|---|---|---|
| Caspar Wistar | 1824 | 1826 | 2 years. |
| Caspar Morris | 1824 | 1827 | 2 years. |
| John Rodman Paul | 1825 | 1826 | 5 months. |
| Charles Mifflin | 1826 | 1828 | 2 years. |
| James A. Washington | 1827 | 1829 | 2 years. |
| George Fox | 1828 | 1830 | 2 years. |
| Ralph Hammersly | 1829 | 1830 | 1 y'r and 3 mo's (died). |
| Thomas Stewardson, Jr. | 1830 | 1832 | 2 years. |
| George W. Norris | 1830 | 1833 | 3 years. |
| Mifflin Wistar | 1832 | 1834 | 2 years. |
| Thomas S. Kirkbride | 1833 | 1835 | 2 years. |
| William W. Gerhard | 1834 | 1836 | 2 years. |
| James A. McCrea | 1835 | 1837 | 2 years. |
| Joshua M. Wallace | 1836 | 1838 | 2 years. |
| Henry H. Smith | 1837 | 1839 | 2 years. |
| John F. Meigs | 1838 | 1840 | 2 years. |
| Alfred Stillé | 1839 | 1841 | 2 years. |
| Anthony E. Stocker | 1840 | 1842 | 2 years. |
| Edward Hartshorne | 1841 | 1843 | 2 years. |
| Moore Robinson | 1842 | 1842 | 8 months (died). |
| Samuel Hollingsworth | 1842 | 1843 | 5 months. |
| Ellerslie Wallace | 1843 | 1844 | 1 year. |
| Fitzwilliam Sargent | 1843 | 1845 | 2 years. |
| John D. Logan | 1844 | 1846 | 2 years. |
| Robert P. Harris | 1845 | 1847 | 2 years. |
| Henry Hartshorne | 1846 | 1848 | 2 years. |
| Wm. McKennan Morgan | 1847 | 1848 | 1 year and 4 months. |
| Spencer Sergeant | 1848 | 1850 | 2 years. |
| Moreton Stillé | 1848 | 1849 | 8 months. |
| James J. Levick | 1849 | 1851 | 2 years and 3 months. |
| Francis W. Lewis | 1849 | 1850 | 1 year. |
| Wm. H. Gobrecht | 1850 | 1851 | 1 year. |
| William Hunt | 1850 | 1852 | 2 years. |
| Addinell Hewson | 1851 | 1852 | 1 year and 6 months. |
| Richard A. F. Penrose | 1851 | 1853 | 2 years. |
| Thomas Hewson Bache | 1852 | 1853 | 1 year and 6 months. |
| James E. Rhoads | 1852 | 1854 | 1 year and 4 months. |
| James Darrach | 1853 | 1854 | 1 year and 6 months. |
| William S. Forbes | 1853 | 1855 | 1 year and 6 months. |
| W. Rush Dunton | 1854 | 1855 | 1 year and 8 months. |
| Augustus Wilson | 1854 | 1856 | 1 year and 6 months. |
| John H. Packard | 1855 | 1856 | 1 year and 6 months. |
| Andrew Fleming | 1855 | 1857 | 1 year and 5 months. |
| Douglass A. Hall | 1856 | 1857 | 1 year and 6 months. |
| George H. Humphreys | 1856 | 1858 | 1 year and 6 months. |

|  | From. | To | Served. |
|---|---|---|---|
| Thomas Geo. Morton | 1857 | 1858 | 1 year and 4 months. |
| Wm. Lehman Wells | 1857 | 1857 | 2 months. |
| Albert H. Smith | 1857 | 1859 | 1 year and 4 months. |
| James H. Hutchinson | 1858 | 1859 | 1 year and 6 months. |
| H. Lenox Hodge | 1858 | 1860 | 1 year and 9 months. |
| George Harlan | 1859 | 1860 | 1 year and 6 months. |
| Thomas B. Reed | 1859 | 1861 | 1 year and 6 months. |
| Edward Livezey | 1859 | 1861 | 1 year and 6 months. |
| Charles A. McCall | 1860 | 1861 | 9 months. |
| Charles Carroll Lee | 1861 | 1862 | 1 year and 6 months. |
| John Ashhurst | 1861 | 1862 | 9 months. |
| William F. Norris | 1861 | 1863 | 1 year and 6 months. |
| William Savery | 1862 | 1863 | 1 year and 6 months. |
| Joseph G. Richardson | 1862 | 1863 | 9 months. |
| Horatio C. Wood, Jr. | 1863 | 1864 | 11 months. |
| William Elmer, Jr. | 1864 | 1864 | 7 months. |
| James Tyson | 1863 | 1864 | 8 months. |
| Thomas Wistar | 1863 | 1864 | 1 year and 6 months. |
| Edward Rhoads | 1864 | 1865 | 1 year and 6 months. |
| T. Hollingsw'th Andrews | 1864 | 1866 | 1 year and 6 months. |
| William Pepper, Jr. | 1865 | 1866 | 1 year and 6 months. |
| Horace Williams | 1865 | 1867 | 1 year and 6 months. |
| Theodore Herbert | 1866 | 1867 | 1 year and 1 month. |
| Horace Binney Hare | 1866 | 1867 | 9 months. |
| James Markoe | 1867 | 1868 | 1 year and 6 months. |
| Herbert Norris | 1867 | 1868 | 1 year and 5 months. |
| Henry Chapman | 1867 | 1869 | 2 years. |
| Elliot Richardson | 1868 | 1870 | 1 year and 6 months. |
| Charles M. Ritz | 1868 | 1869 | 1 year. |
| Charles T. Hunter | 1869 | 1870 | 1 year. |
| Arthur Van Harlingen | 1869 | 1871 | 1 year and 6 months. |
| Morris Longstreth | 1870 | 1871 | 1 year and 6 months. |
| James C. Wilson | 1870 | 1871 | 1 year. |
| Robert H. Alison | 1871 | 1872 | 1 year and 6 months. |
| George S. Gerhard | 1871 | 1872 | 10 months. |
| Daniel Bray | 1871 | 1872 | 6 months. |
| William C. Cox | 1872 | 1873 | 1 year and 6 months. |
| Arthur V. Meigs | 1872 | 1874 | 1 year and 6 months. |
| Ewing Jordan | 1872 | 1873 | 7 months. |
| Frank Woodbury | 1873 | 1874 | 1 year. |
| Edward W. Jameson | 1873 | 1875 | 1 year and 4 months. |
| J. Aubrey Lippincott | 1873 | 1875 | 1 year and 6 months. |
| Morris J. Lewis | 1874 | 1875 | 1 year and 6 months. |
| T. Hewson Bradford | 1875 | 1876 | 1 year and 8 months. |
| John B. Roberts | 1875 |  |  |
| Wm. Barton Hopkins | 1875 |  |  |
| M. Frank Kirkbride | 1876 |  |  |

## APOTHECARIES.

| | From. | To. | Served. |
|---|---|---|---|
| Jonathan Roberts | 1752 | 1755 | 2 years and 4 months. |
| John Morgan | 1755 | 1756 | 1 year and 1 month. |
| John Bond | 1756 | 1758 | 2 years. |
| James A. Bayard | 1758 | 1759 | 1 year. |
| John Davis | 1767 | 1768 | 7 months. |
| William Smith | 1770 | 1773 | 2 years and 10 months. |
| Thomas Boulter | 1773 | 1773 | 2 months. |
| James Hutchinson | 1773 | 1775 | 2 years and 1 month. |
| James Dunlap | 1775 | 1776 | 1 year. |
| Peter Yarnall | 1780 | 1781 | 1 year and 5 months. |
| Gustavus F. Kielman | 1781 | 1782 | 1 year and 4 months. |
| James Hartley | 1782 | 1784 | 1 year and 3 months. |
| *Nicholas B. Waters | 1784 | 1787 | 3 years and 1 month. |
| Graham Hoskins | 1821 | 1823 | 2 years. |
| Robert Harris | 1823 | 1824 | 10 months. |
| Samuel C. Sheppard | 1824 | 1825 | 1 year and 2 months. |
| Newberry Smith, Jr. | 1825 | 1829 | 4 years. |
| Franklin R. Smith | 1829 | 1831 | 2 years. |
| John Conrad | 1831 | 1870 | 39 years. |
| Jacob K. Hecker | 1870 | 1874 | 4 years and 2 months. |
| Jacob K. Hecker | 1876 | | |
| Charles Wirgman | 1874 | 1876 | 2 years and 3 months. |

\* From 1787 to 1821, the duties of the Apothecary were performed by the Medical Apprentices.

## III.

## STEWARDS AND MATRONS OF THE HOSPITAL.

| Stewards. | From. | To. | Served |
|---|---|---|---|
| Matthew Taylor | 1758 | 1759 | 1 year. |
| *George Weed | 1760 | 1767 | 7 years and 3 months. |
| *Robert Slade | 1768 | 1769 | 1 y'r and 2 mo's (died). |
| John Saxton | 1773 | 1776 | 3 years. |
| *John Story | 1776 | 1780 | 4 years. |
| Joseph Henszey | 1780 | 1796 | 16 years. |
| Francis Higgins | {1796 1808} | {1803 1813} | 12 years and 3 months (died). |
| William Johnston | 1803 | 1808 | 4 years and 8 months. |
| Samuel Mason | 1813 | 1826 | 13 years. |
| Isaac Bonsall | 1826 | 1830 | 4 years and 6 months. |
| Allen Clapp | 1830 | 1849 | 18 years and 9 months. |
| William G. Malin | 1849 | | |

| Matrons. | From. | To. | Served. |
|---|---|---|---|
| †Elizabeth Gardner | 1751 | 1760 | 9 years. |
| Esther Weed | 1760 | 1767 | 6 y'rs and 8 mo's (died). |
| †Mary Ball | 1767 | 1768 | 1 year and 5 months. |
| †Sarah Harlan | 1768 | 1772 | 4 y'rs and 5 mo's (died). |
| Sophia Saxton | 1773 | 1776 | 3 years. |
| Mary Story | 1776 | 1780 | 4 years. |
| Deborah Henszey | 1780 | 1790 | 10 years and 3 months |
| Mary Falconer | 1790 | 1795 | 5 years.    [(died). |
| Ann Henszey | 1795 | 1796 | 9 months. |
| Hannah Higgins | {1796 1808} | {1803 1813} | 12 years and 3 months. |
| Abigail Johnston | 1803 | 1808 | 4 years and 8 months. |
| Mary Mason | 1813 | 1826 | 13 years. |
| Ann Bonsall | 1826 | 1830 | 4 y'rs and 3 mo's (died). |
| Margaret Clapp | 1830 | 1835 | 4 y'rs and 5 mo's (died). |
| Margaret Robinson | 1835 | 1835 | 4 months. |
| Elizabeth Clapp | 1835 | 1842 | 6 years and 10 months. |
| Elizabeth Hooton | 1842 | 1848 | 6 years. |
| Harriet P. Smith | 1848 | 1853 | 5 years and 4 months. |
| Mary D. Sharpless | 1853 | 1876 | 23 years. |
| Anna M. Morris | 1876 | | |

\* These also acted as Apothecaries.
† These ladies acted also as Stewards.

## IV.

*The following table exhibits the number of pay and poor patients, and the total number admitted into the Pennsylvania Hospital in the City, and the average number maintained during each year from its foundation to 4th mo. (April) 22, 1876.*

|  | Year. | Pay. | Poor. | Total. | Average. |
|---|---|---|---|---|---|
| Admitted from Feb. 11th, 1752, to end of April, | 1753 | 24 | 40 | 64 | 9 |
|  | 1754 | 14 | 39 | 53 | 12 |
|  | 1755 | 13 | 60 | 73 | 17 |
|  | 1756 | 7 | 61 | 78 | 17 |
|  | 1757 | 13 | 68 | 81 | 17 |
|  | 1758 | 29 | 85 | 114 | 33 |
|  | 1759 | 25 | 102 | 127 | 34 |
|  | 1760 | 32 | 105 | 137 | 40 |
|  | 1761 | 40 | 113 | 153 | 45 |
|  | 1762 | 29 | 128 | 157 | 47 |
|  | 1763 | 46 | 194 | 240 | 73 |
|  | 1764 | 50 | 272 | 322 | 101 |
|  | 1765 | 45 | 261 | 306 | 111 |
|  | 1766 | 56 | 283 | 339 | 119 |
|  | 1767 | 38 | 307 | 345 | 120 |
|  | 1768 | 54 | 337 | 391 | 123 |
|  | 1769 | 32 | 353 | 385 | 110 |
|  | 1770 | 49 | 336 | 385 | 113 |
|  | 1771 | 44 | 338 | 382 | 118 |
|  | 1772 | 44 | 349 | 393 | 117 |
|  | 1773 | 46 | 315 | 361 | 105 |
|  | 1774 | 63 | 374 | 437 | 117 |
|  | 1775 | 60 | 361 | 421 | 105 |
|  | 1776 | 42 | 393 | 435 | 89 |
|  | 1777 | 109 | 268 | 377 | 67 |
|  | 1778 | 31 | 96 | 127 | 39 |
|  | 1779 | 16 | 107 | 123 | 36 |
|  | 1780 | 10 | 118 | 128 | 35 |
|  | 1781 | 18 | 103 | 121 | 35 |
|  | 1782 | 69 | 42 | 111 | 36 |
|  | 1783 | 83 | 23 | 106 | 37 |
|  | 1784 | 156 | 47 | 203 | 61 |
|  | 1785 | 133 | 35 | 168 | 51 |
|  | 1786 | 113 | 25 | 138 | 51 |
|  | 1787 | 108 | 30 | 138 | 54 |

| Year. | Pay. | Poor. | Total. | Average. |
|---|---|---|---|---|
| 1788 | 78 | 32 | 110 | 54 |
| 1789 | 49 | 28 | 77 | 47 |
| 1790 | 51 | 27 | 78 | 46 |
| 1791 | 73 | 32 | 105 | 52 |
| 1792 | 107 | 72 | 179 | 64 |
| 1793 | 87 | 63 | 150 | 63 |
| 1794 | 170 | 78 | 248 | 71 |
| 1795 | 107 | 67 | 174 | 72 |
| 1796 | 113 | 103 | 216 | 69 |
| 1797 | 114 | 89 | 203 | 75 |
| 1798 | 101 | 71 | 172 | 78 |
| 1799 | 60 | 66 | 126 | 74 |
| 1800 | 80 | 96 | 176 | 78 |
| 1801 | 106 | 70 | 176 | 85 |
| 1802 | 176 | 73 | 249 | 87 |
| 1803 | 217 | 87 | 304 | 114 |
| 1804 | 214 | 88 | 302 | 113 |
| 1805 | 231 | 89 | 320 | 103 |
| 1806 | 241 | 98 | 339 | 109 |
| 1807 | 338 | 115 | 453 | 129 |
| 1808 | 288 | 121 | 409 | 122 |
| 1809 | 419 | 141 | 560 | 158 |
| 1810 | 216 | 152 | 368 | 127 |
| 1811 | 281 | 171 | 452 | 138 |
| 1812 | 373 | 172 | 545 | 150 |
| 1813 | 376 | 145 | 521 | 161 |
| 1814 | 307 | 140 | 447 | 163 |
| 1815 | 235 | 159 | 394 | 147 |
| 1816 | 500 | 181 | 681 | 178 |
| 1817 | 483 | 201 | 684 | 200 |
| 1818 | 468 | 170 | 638 | 199 |
| 1819 | 474 | 243 | 717 | 214 |
| 1820 | 457 | 292 | 749 | 226 |
| 1821 | 414 | 286 | 700 | 208 |
| 1822 | 300 | 244 | 544 | 158 |
| 1823 | 346 | 342 | 688 | 170 |
| 1824 | 363 | 384 | 747 | 178 |
| 1825 | 353 | 391 | 744 | 177 |
| 1826 | 368 | 362 | 730 | 175 |
| 1827 | 416 | 383 | 809 | 183 |
| 1828 | 427 | 460 | 887 | 202 |
| 1829 | 492 | 658 | 1150 | 219 |
| 1830 | 455 | 675 | 1130 | 225 |
| 1831 | 506 | 616 | 1112 | 233 |
| 1832 | 552 | 587 | 1139 | 249 |
| 1833 | 455 | 587 | 1042 | 232 |
| 1834 | 394 | 589 | 983 | 228 |
| 1835 | 345 | 644 | 989 | 236 |

| Year. | Pay. | Poor. | Total. | Average. |
|---|---|---|---|---|
| 1836 | 390 | 615 | 1005 | 227 |
| 1837 | 382 | 592 | 974 | 213 |
| 1838 | 382 | 655 | 1037 | 202 |
| 1839 | 333 | 638 | 971 | 210 |
| 1840 | 290 | 660 | 950 | 215 |
| 1841 | 328 | 571 | 899 | 196 |
| 1842 | 321 | 503 | 824 | 106* |
| 1843 | 328 | 577 | 805 | 93 |
| 1844 | 271 | 667 | 938 | 101 |
| 1845 | 267 | 688 | 955 | 102 |
| 1846 | 265 | 808 | 1073 | 114 |
| 1847 | 335 | 942 | 1277 | 127 |
| 1848 | 478 | 1068 | 1546 | 142 |
| 1849 | 526 | 1126 | 1652 | 148 |
| 1850 | 565 | 1250 | 1815 | 159 |
| 1851 | 467 | 1298 | 1765 | 158 |
| 1852 | 506 | 1140 | 1646 | 144 |
| 1853 | 543 | 1164 | 1707 | 162 |
| 1854 | 591 | 1240 | 1831 | 174 |
| 1855 | 621 | 1275 | 1896 | 178 |
| 1856 | 560 | 1154 | 1714 | 158 |
| 1857 | 614 | 1066 | 1680 | 159 |
| 1858 | 530 | 1126 | 1656 | 162 |
| 1859 | 511 | 1147 | 1658 | 164 |
| 1860 | 623 | 1173 | 1796 | 172 |
| 1861 | 651 | 1191 | 1842 | 180 |
| 1862 | 530 | 1148 | 1678 | 166 |
| 1863 | 606 | 1004 | 1610 | 183 |
| 1864 | 453 | 1287 | 1740 | 155 |
| 1865 | 441 | 1397 | 1838 | 157 |
| 1866 | 491 | 1509 | 2000 | 167 |
| 1867 | 435 | 1338 | 1773 | 170 |
| 1868 | 421 | 1366 | 1787 | 168 |
| 1869 | 416 | 1532 | 1948 | 160 |
| 1870 | 338 | 1410 | 1748 | 153 |
| 1871 | 329 | 1605 | 1934 | 170 |
| 1872 | 406 | 1599 | 2005 | 176 |
| 1873 | 441 | 1563 | 2004 | 155 |
| 1874 | 459 | 1328 | 1787 | 146 |
| 1875 | 488 | 1328 | 1816 | 162 |
| 1876 | 368 | 1270 | 1638 | 159 |

* This reduction in the average population of the Hospital was caused by the removal, in 1841, of more than 90 insane patients (mostly permanent boarders) to the Pennsylvania Hospital for the Insane.

Since the establishment of the Hospital in 1752, there have been admitted into it 95,848 patients, of whom 62,357 have been poor persons, supported at the expense of the Institution. Of these 95,848 patients there have been

| | |
|---|---:|
| Cured | 61,880 |
| Relieved | 12,849 |
| Discharged without material improvement | 7,295 |
| Discharged for misconduct or eloped | 2,105 |
| Pregnant women safely delivered | 1,335 |
| Infants born in the Hospital and discharged in health | 1,255 |
| Died | 8,974 |
| | 95,693 |
| Remaining Fourth month 22d, 1876 | 155 |
| | 95,848 |

In addition to those above enumerated, 15,258 persons were attended as *out-patients*, and furnished with medicine at the expense of the Hospital. This was done during the years 1797 to 1817, when, in consequence of the establishment of institutions having this special object, the dispensary practice of the Hospital was discontinued. The out-door department was resumed 11th mo. 1st, 1872, and from that date to 5th mo. 2d, 1876, 9327 were admitted—thus making altogether 24,585 patients treated in this department.

## V.
## OFFICERS OF THE INSTITUTION.
### ELECTED BY THE CONTRIBUTORS.

At the 125th Annual Meeting of this Corporation, held 5th month 1st, 1876, the following Contributors were elected for the ensuing year:—

### MANAGERS.

WILLIAM BIDDLE,  
ALEX. J. DERBYSHIRE,  
SAMUEL MASON,  
SAMUEL WELSH,  
WISTAR MORRIS,  
JACOB P. JONES,  
BENJAMIN H. SHOEMAKER,  
ALEXANDER BIDDLE,  
JOSEPH B. TOWNSEND,  
JOSEPH C. TURNPENNY,  
T. WISTAR BROWN,  
HENRY HAINES.

### TREASURER.
JOHN T. LEWIS.

## APPOINTED BY THE MANAGERS.
### HOSPITAL ON PINE STREET.

STEWARD, WILLIAM G. MALIN.

MATRON, ———————

ASSISTANT MATRON, FANNIE G. IRWIN.

CLERK, LIBRARIAN, AND ASSISTANT STEWARD, JONATHAN RICHARDS.

APOTHECARY, CHARLES WIRGMAN.

### PHYSICIANS.
JOHN FORSYTH MEIGS, M.D.,  
JACOB M. DA COSTA, M.D,  
JAMES H. HUTCHINSON, M.D.,  
J. AITKEN MEIGS, M.D.

### SURGEONS.
ADDINELL HEWSON, M.D.,  
WILLIAM HUNT, M.D.,  
THOS. GEORGE MORTON, M.D.,  
RICHARD J. LEVIS, M.D.

### RESIDENT PHYSICIANS.
T. HEWSON BRADFORD, M.D.,  
WM. BARTON HOPKINS, M.D.,  
JOHN B. ROBERTS, M.D.

PATHOLOGIST AND CURATOR, MORRIS LONGSTRETH, M.D.

PATHOLOGICAL CHEMIST, HORACE BINNEY HARE, M.D.

MICROSCOPIST, JOSEPH G. RICHARDSON, M.D.

### OUT-PATIENT DEPARTMENT.
#### PHYSICIANS.
MORRIS LONGSTRETH, M.D.,  
JOSEPH G. RICHARDSON, M.D.,  
JOSEPH J. KIRKBRIDE, M.D.

#### SURGEONS.
CHARLES HUNTER, M.D.,  
THOMAS H. ANDREWS, M.D.,  
ELLIOTT RICHARDSON, M.D.,  
WILLIAM ASHBRIDGE, M.D.

## VI.

## PENNSYLVANIA HOSPITAL FOR THE INSANE.

The Pennsylvania Hospital for the Insane (situated in West Philadelphia) was opened for the reception of patients on the 1st day of the year 1841, since which time there have been admitted into it—

| Males. | Females. | Pay. | Free. | Total. |
|---|---|---|---|---|
| 3831 | 3336 | 5635 | 1532 | 7167 |

Of the whole number admitted have been discharged—

| | |
|---|---|
| Cured . . . . . . | 3324 |
| Much improved . . . . | } 1677 |
| Improved . . . . . | |
| Stationary . . . . . . | 853 |
| Died . . . . . . | 894 |
| | 6748 |
| Remain under treatment | 419 |
| Total, | 7167 |

The following table exhibits the gradual increase in number of insane patients in the Hospital, being the number under care at the close of each official year since it was opened.

| At the close of the year ending 4th mo. 24, | | | | Average number during the year. |
|---|---|---|---|---|
| | 1841 there were | 97 patients. | | |
| " | 1842 " | 109 | " | 106 |
| " | 1843 " | 135 | " | 120 |
| " | 1844 " | 147 | " | 138 |
| " | 1845 " | 158 | " | 154 |
| " | 1846 " | 180 | " | 169 |
| " | 1847 " | 188 | " | 172 |
| " | 1848 " | 202 | " | 192 |
| " | 1849 " | 208 | " | 202 |
| " | 1850 " | 230 | " | 210 |
| " | 1851 " | 230 | " | 216 |
| " | 1852 " | 227 | " | 226 |
| " | 1853 " | 226 | " | 223 |
| " | 1854 " | 229 | " | 232 |
| " | 1855 " | 236 | " | 228 |
| " | 1856 " | 230 | " | 234 |
| " | 1857 " | 243 | " | 234 |

|  |  |  |  | Average number during the year. |
|---|---|---|---|---|
| At the close of the year ending 4th mo. 24, | 1858 there were 235 patients. | | | 237 |
| " | 1859 | " | 252 | " | 239 |
| " | 1860 | " | 264 | " | 256 |
| " | 1861 | " | 277 | " | 276 |
| " | 1862 | " | 265 | " | 272 |
| " | 1863 | " | 272 | " | 273 |
| " | 1864 | " | 290 | " | 286 |
| " | 1865 | " | 297 | " | 288 |
| " | 1866 | " | 319 | " | 305 |
| " | 1867 | " | 336 | " | 311 |
| " | 1868 | " | 361 | " | 349 |
| " | 1869 | " | 337 | " | 346 |
| " | 1870 | " | 331 | " | 326 |
| " | 1871 | " | 356 | " | 352 |
| " | 1872 | " | 398 | " | 385 |
| " | 1873 | " | 391 | " | 404 |
| " | 1874 | " | 426 | " | 412 |
| " | 1875 | " | 434 | " | 424 |
| " | 1876 | " | 427 | " | 433 |

The total number of patients treated for insanity in both branches of the Pennsylvania Hospital since its foundation in 1752 is 11,507.

## PHYSICIAN-IN-CHIEF AND SUPERINTENDENT,
### Dr. THOMAS S. KIRKBRIDE (Elected 1840).

#### ASSISTANT PHYSICIANS.

|  | From. | To. |  |
|---|---|---|---|
| Dr. Edward Hartshorne | 1840 | 1841 | 3 months. |
| " Francis Gurney Smith | 1841 | 1841 | 9 months. |
| " Robert A. Given | 1842 | 1844 | 2 years and 4 months. |
| " John Curwen | 1844 | 1849 | 5 years and 4 months. |
| " Thomas J. Mendenhall | 1849 | 1851 | 1 year and 4 months. |
| " J. Edwards Lee | {1851, 1862} | {1856, 1868} | 11 years and 7 months. |
| " Edward A. Smith | 1856 | 1862 | 6 years and 1 month. |
| " William P. Moon | 1868 |  |  |
| " Rob't J. Hess, 2d Ass't | 1875 |  |  |

**MALE DEPARTMENT.**

| | | | |
|---|---|---|---|
| Dr. S. Preston Jones, 1st As't | 1859 | | |

**2D ASSISTANTS.**

| | From | To | |
|---|---|---|---|
| Dr. William Longshore | 1860 | 1862 | 1 year and 7 months. |
| " James Hall | 1863 | 1863 | 6 months. |
| " Daniel Beitler | 1864 | 1867 | 3 years and 2 months. |
| " John T Wilson | 1867 | 1868 | 1 year and 2 months. |
| " J. Roe Bradner | 1869 | 1871 | 2 years and 5 months. |
| " William H. Bartles | 1871 | | |
| " Frank G. Corson, 3d As't | 1875 | | |

#### STEWARDS AND MATRONS OF THE HOSPITAL FOR THE INSANE.

| Stewards. | From. | To. | Served. |
|---|---|---|---|
| William G. Malin | 1840 | 1849 | 8 years and 8 months. |
| Jonathan Richards | {1849, 1859} | {1853, 1869} | 14 years and 2 months. |
| John Wistar | 1853 | 1866 | 13 years. |
| Joshua P. Edge | 1866 | 1873 | 6 years and 2 months. |
| Joseph Jones | 1870 | | |
| George Jones | 1873 | | |
| **Matrons.** | | | |
| Mary D. Sharpless | 1840 | 1849 | 8 years and 6 months. |
| Margaret C. Richards | {1849, 1859} | {1853, 1865} | 9 years and 9 months. |
| Margaret N. Wistar | 1853 | 1866 | 13 years. |
| Harriet P. Smith | 1865 | 1870 | 5 years. |
| Jane Mitchell | 1866 | 1867 | 1 year and 1 month. |
| Anne Jones | 1870 | | |

## VII.
## OFFICERS OF THE INSTITUTION
### FOR THE DEPARTMENT OF THE INSANE.

#### MANAGERS.

| | |
|---|---|
| WILLIAM BIDDLE, *President.* | JACOB P. JONES, |
| BENJ. H. SHOEMAKER, *Secretary.* | ALEXANDER BIDDLE, |
| A. J. DERBYSHIRE, | JOSEPH B. TOWNSEND, |
| SAMUEL MASON, | JOSEPH C. TURNPENNY, |
| SAMUEL WELSH, | T. WISTAR BROWN, |
| WISTAR MORRIS, | HENRY HAINES. |

#### TREASURER.
JOHN T. LEWIS.

#### PHYSICIAN IN CHIEF AND SUPERINTENDENT.
THOMAS S. KIRKBRIDE, M.D.

| Department for Males. | Department for Females. |
|---|---|
| ASSISTANT PHYSICIAN. | ASSISTANT PHYSICIAN. |
| S. PRESTON JONES, M.D. | WILLIAM P. MOON, M.D. |
| 2D ASSISTANT PHYSICIAN. | 2D ASSISTANT PHYSICIAN. |
| WM. H. BARTLES, M.D. | ROBERT J. HESS, M.D. |
| 3D ASSISTANT PHYSICIAN. | |
| FRANK F. CORSON, M.D. | STEWARD. |
| STEWARD. | JOSEPH JONES. |
| GEORGE JONES. | |
| MATRON. | MATRON. |
| HANNAH P. SAGER. | ANNE JONES. |

## VIII.

## LEGACIES

BEQUEATHED TO THE PENNSYLVANIA HOSPITAL
FROM 1751 TO 1876.

### A.

| Year | Name | Amount |
|---|---|---|
| 1761 | Mary Allen, mother of Chief Justice Allen | $266 66 |
| " | Mary Andrews, ground rents valued at | 533 33 |
| " | Margaret Asheton | 26 67 |
| 1765 | Hannah Allen | 26 67 |
| 1770 | Robert Allison, Lancaster County | 266 66 |
| 1775 | Enoch Abrahams, Radnor | 53 33 |
| 1776 | Aaron Ashbridge | 80 00 |
| 1777 | Caleb Ash, butcher | 31 33 |
| 1803 | Caleb Ash | 200 00 |
| 1812 | Susanna P. Abington | 250 00 |
| 1816 | George Aston | 400 00 |
| 1873 | John Agnew | 1425 00 |

### B.

| Year | Name | | | Amount |
|---|---|---|---|---|
| 1761 | John Baldwin | | | 133 33 |
| 1765 | William Bromwich | | | 53 33 |
| " | George Benzel | | | 80 00 |
| " | General Henry Bouquet | | | 106 66 |
| " | Christopher Brown, Queen Ann's Co., Maryland (received from 1765 to 1776) | | | 1333 33 |
| 1776 | Daniel Bornemann, Philadelphia Co. | | | 16 00 |
| 1770 | James Bright, hatter | | | 80 00 |
| 1773 | William Bettle | | | 66 66 |
| 1807 | John Blakey | | | 266 66 |
| 1843 | Pierre Antoine Bleuon (received from 1843 to 1851) | | | 1,700 00 |
| 1849 | Paul Beck, Jr. | | | 975 00 |
| 1860 | Benjamin F. Butler | 500 00 | | |
| 1862 | "    "    " | 150 00 | | |
| 1870 | "    "    " | | 150 00 | 800 00 |
| 1863 | Samuel Breck | | | 225 62 |
| 1869 | Isaac Barton | | | 4,300 00 |
| 1872 | Nathan Barrett | | | 95 00 |

## C.

| | | | | |
|---|---|---|---|---|
| 1755 | Joshua Crosby | | $266 | 66 |
| 1760 | Henry Croyder, Lancaster Co. | £20 0 0 ⎫ | 100 | 89 |
| 1762 | "        "        " | 17 16 9 ⎭ | | |
| 1761 | Rebecca Cooper | | 53 | 30 |
| 1765 | Thomas Campbell | | 26 | 67 |
| 1769 | William Coleman, Esq. | | 133 | 33 |
| 1772 | Charles Cress | | 400 | 00 |
| 1773 | John Roberts Cadwalader, of Whitpain | | 13 | 33 |
| 1785 | Deborah Claypole, £6 per annum | | 266 | 66 |
| 1806 | Samuel Cooper, M.D. (received from 1806 to 1812) | | 2,415 | 76 |
| 1814 | William Chancellor | | 1,000 | 00 |
| 1817 | Hannah Clarke | | 50 | 00 |
| 1819 | Nathaniel Curren | | 133 | 33 |
| 1821 | Robert Correy | | 500 | 00 |
| 1857 | Jasper Cope | | 5,000 | 00 |
| 1858 | Elliott Cresson | | 5,728 | 84 |
| 1859 | Jane Clark | | 1,000 | 00 |
| 1863 | John Clark | | 95 | 00 |
| 1870 | Cozzens | 423 98 | | |
| 1872 | " | 33 33 | 457 | 31 |
| 1874 | Esther L. Cooper | | 2,000 | 00 |
| "    | St. George Tucker Campbell | | 1,000 | 00 |

## D.

| | | | |
|---|---|---|---|
| 1761 | Peter Dicks | 133 | 33 |
| 1766 | Matthew Drason | 66 | 66 |
| 1769 | Peter Delage | 106 | 66 |
| 1770 | Mary Dougherty | 13 | 33 |
| "    | John Davis, of Darby | 133 | 33 |
| 1771 | Gilbert Deacon | 26 | 67 |
| 1774 | Jacob Dubree | 133 | 33 |
| 1782 | Esther Duche | 133 | 33 |
| 1801 | William Dawson, Jr. | 133 | 33 |
| 1820 | William Dawson, brewer | 400 | 00 |
| 1808 | Andrew Doz (received from 1808 to 1844) | 5,028 | 89 |
| 1811 | Christian H. Denckla | 200 | 00 |
| 1812 | John Descamps | 500 | 00 |
| 1820 | Elizabeth Dawson | 100 | 00 |
| 1832 | Dorothy Dale | 390 | 00 |
| 1860 | Josiah Dawson | 11,500 | 00 |
| 1871 | Henry Duhring | 100 | 00 |
| 1863 | F. M. Drexel | 900 | 00 |
| 1873 | Mordecai L. Dawson | 5,000 | 00 |

### E.

| | | | |
|---|---|---:|---:|
| 1767 | Hudson Emlen | $106 | 66 |
| 1771 | Rachel Emlen | 133 | 33 |
| 1775 | Christian Edel | 13 | 33 |
| 1824 | John C. Evans, carpenter | 400 | 00 |
| 1854 | J. Eley | 3,758 | 10 |

### F.

| | | | | | |
|---|---|---:|---:|---:|---:|
| 1790 | Robert Fleming (received 1790 and 1791) | | | 487 | 66 |
| 1800 | Benjamin Fuller | | | 400 | 00 |
| 1808 | Captain Nathaniel Falconer | | | 133 | 33 |
| 1810 | Thomas Fisher | | | 100 | 00 |
| 1815 | Sarah Falconer | | | 80 | 00 |
| 1821 | Anthony Fothergill | | | 100 | 00 |
| 1853 | Robert Fielding | 4,460 | 24 | | |
| 1864 | " " | 239 | 79 | | |
| 1868 | " " | 1,873 | 92 | 6,573 | 95 |
| 1867 | Joseph Fisher | 35,459 | 25 | | |
| 1868 | " " | 9,126 | 18 | 44,585 | 43 |

### G.

| | | | |
|---|---|---:|---:|
| 1762 | Thomas Griffin, of Bucks Co. | 26 | 67 |
| 1765 | Samuel Grubb, of Chester Co. | 133 | 33 |
| 1772 | Isaac Greenleafe | 266 | 69 |
| " | Michael Gross, of Lancaster | 36 | 00 |
| 1808 | Thomas George | 200 | 00 |
| 1817 | Margery Ged | 300 | 00 |
| 1828 | John Grandom | 2,925 | 00 |
| 1832 | Stephen Girard | 29,250 | 00 |
| 1835 | Ann Guest | 487 | 50 |
| 1870 | John W. Grigg | 47,500 | 00 |
| 1871 | James R. Greeves | 950 | 00 |
| 1872 | George W. Groove | 5,000 | 00 |
| 1873 | Jesse George | 20,000 | 00 |

### H.

| | | | |
|---|---|---:|---:|
| 1765 | Elizabeth Hinmarsh | 13 | 33 |
| 1769 | Edward Hill, of Berks Co. | 266 | 66 |
| " | Charles Harrison, of Boston | 2,040 | 00 |
| 1770 | Philip Hulbert | 53 | 33 |
| 1785 | Michael Hutchison | 133 | 33 |
| 1795 | Reuben Haines | 266 | 66 |
| " | Margaret Haines | 266 | 66 |
| 1813 | Samuel Howell | 266 | 66 |

| | | | |
|---|---|---|---:|
| 1815 | Isaac Harvey | | $1,200 00 |
| 1822 | Josiah Hewes | | 1,200 00 |
| 1824 | Godfrey Haga | | 1,000 00 |
| 1836 | Elizabeth Hampton | | 61 25 |
| 1866 | Mary Ann Harris | | 800 00 |
| 1867 | John Harding, Jr. | | 1,000 00 |

## I & J.

| | | |
|---|---|---:|
| 1768 | Richard Johnson | 133 33 |
| 1770 | Mary Jacob | 26 67 |
| 1869 | N. S. Jennings | 120 00 |

## K.

| | | | |
|---|---|---:|---:|
| 1772 | Conrad Kelmer | | 26 67 |
| 1801 | Peter Knight | | 533 33 |
| 1803 | Robert Knox, mariner | | 266 66 |
| 1808 | John Keble (received from 1808 to 1851) | | 26,914 17 |
| 1854 | John Keble | 430 54 | |
| 1855 | "          " | 607 02 | 1,037 56 |
| 1871 | William Kirkham | | 100 00 |

## L.

| | | |
|---|---|---:|
| 1775 | Jacob Lewis, a ground rent, value | 225 00 |
| 1776 | William Logan | 266 66 |
| 1778 | Mary Loveday | 133 33 |
| 1782 | Joseph Lownes | 26 67 |
| 1795 | Samuel Lewis | 266 66 |
| 1796 | Hannah Lownes | 26 67 |
| 1800 | Mordecai Lewis | 266 66 |
| 1803 | James Logan, merchant | 1,333 33 |
| 1805 | Christopher Ludwig | 266 66 |
| 1823 | Josiah H. Lownes | 500 00 |
| 1835 | Mahlon Lawrence | 292 50 |
| 1870 | Margaret Latimer | 5,000 00 |

## M.

| | | |
|---|---|---:|
| 1762 | James McCulloch | 23 91 |
| 1765 | Samuel Mickle | 66 66 |
| "    " | Joseph Marshall | 133 33 |
| 1766 | Frederick Mirele, Springfield, Phila. Co. | 29 46 |
| 1768 | Daniel Murphy | 8 00 |
| 1774 | Archibald McLean | 26 67 |
| 1774 | Samuel Morton | 133 33 |
| 1776 | Sarah Morris | 66 66 |

8

| | | | | |
|---|---|---|---|---|
| 1778 | William Mitchell | | $133 | 33 |
| 1789 | Robert Morton | | 133 | 33 |
| 1791 | Lucea McCalla | | 88 | 87 |
| 1794 | Alexander Major, of Gwynedd | | 26 | 67 |
| 1800 | Deborah Morris (ground rent, per annum $73 33) | | 1,222 | 00 |
| 1801 | Patrick McGuier, schoolmaster | | 278 | 50 |
| 1804 | Mary Morris | | 133 | 33 |
| 1813 | Sarah Moore | | 1,215 | 00 |
| 1816 | Sarah Marriott | | 66 | 66 |
| " | Robert Montgomery | | 1,000 | 00 |
| 1821 | Rachel McCulloch | | 26 | 67 |
| 1823 | Moses B. Moody (received from 1823 to 1826) | | 1,559 | 40 |
| 1844 | John Murray | | 50 | 00 |
| 1855 | Jacob G. Morris | | 507 | 50 |
| 1859 | Abram Miller | 1,000 00 | | |
| 1860 | "        " | 2,559 73 | | |
| 1863 | "        " | 12,833 33 | 16,393 | 06 |
| 1860 | Catharine Morris | | 190 | 00 |
| 1871 | Benjamin Marshall | | 1,000 | 00 |
| " | Samuel V. Merrick | | 250 | 00 |

N.

| | | | |
|---|---|---|---|
| 1763 | Content Nicholson | 66 | 66 |
| 1769 | Isaac Norris | 266 | 66 |
| 1774 | Samuel Neave | 1,033 | 33 |
| 1792 | Thomas Nedrow | 66 | 66 |
| 1807 | Charles Nicholes | 5,000 | 00 |
| 1868 | Abram J. Nunes | 3,225 | 12 |
| 1872 | Charles Norton | 200 | 00 |

O.

| | | | |
|---|---|---|---|
| 1767 | George Owen | 133 | 33 |
| 1772 | Ann Opertony | 168 | 75 |
| 1870 | George Ord | 25,730 | 68 |

P.

| | | | |
|---|---|---|---|
| 1754 | Mary Plumstead | 133 | 33 |
| 1771 | John Peters | 26 | 67 |
| 1776 | Meriam Potts | 23 | 67 |
| 1791 | Sarah Parrock | 800 | 00 |
| 1792 | Esther Pemberton | 133 | 33 |
| 1796 | Thomas Paschall | 106 | 66 |
| " | John Pennell | 66 | 66 |
| 1813 | John Pemberton | 133 | 33 |
| 1828 | Martha Powell | 585 | 00 |

| | | | |
|---|---|---|---|
| 7834 | Elliston Perot | | $100 00 |
| 1840 | John Perot | | 100 00 |
| 1848 | Joseph Price | | 1,000 00 |
| 1852 | John Pea | | 1,457 57 |
| 1855 | John Paul | | 975 00 |
| 1861 | Jos. Price, Exr. of S. R. Simmons | | 5,000 00 |
| 1864 | Hannah Parke, Exr. of | | 3,800 00 |
| " | Francis Pierpont, Exrs. of | 2,700 00 | |
| 1865 | "       "       " | 1,134 00 | 3,834 00 |
| 1867 | Dr. Casper W. Pennock | | 1,000 00 |
| " | Edward Perot | | 1,000 00 |
| 1870 | Charles Perot | | 1,000 00 |
| " | Sarah Phipps | | 200 00 |
| 1875 | Joseph Pleasants | | 95 00 |

### R.

| | | |
|---|---|---|
| 1761 | Francis Rawle | 133 33 |
| 1765 | Rudman Robeson | 533 33 |
| 1766 | Jacob Rightlinger, Lebanon, Lanc. Co. | 121 93 |
| 1767 | Septimus Robeson | 133 33 |
| 1771 | Thomas Robinson | 133 33 |
| 1774 | William Rakestraw | 53 33 |
| 1796 | Daniel Rundle | 666 66 |
| 1800 | Peter Reeve, mariner | 133 33 |
| 1804 | John Roberts | 133 33 |
| 1809 | Hugh Roberts | 266 66 |
| 1866 | William Richardson | 890 00 |
| 1870 | Evans Rogers | 952 50 |
| 1873 | Edward Roberts | 4,750 00 |

### S.

| | | |
|---|---|---|
| 1758 | Christopher Sauer | 53 33 |
| 1761 | Richard Spring | 98 35 |
| 1766 | Mary Standley | 66 66 |
| " | Christopher Saunderson | 26 66 |
| 1771 | Daniel Stanton | 26 66 |
| " | Joseph Stout | 26 66 |
| 1772 | Ann Strettell | 53 33 |
| 1774 | Samuel Sansom | 80 00 |
| 1792 | Samuel Scott, Lancaster Co. | 81 86 |
| 1794 | James Stoops | 1,889 31 |
| 1798 | Resolve Smith | 533 33 |
| 1799 | Buckridge Sims | 266 66 |
| 1803 | William Sheaff | 300 00 |
| 1811 | Esther Sprague | 848 13 |
| 1827 | Joseph Sansom | 487 50 |
| 1829 | Samuel Scotten | 196 67 |
| 1830 | Paul Siemen | 1,950 00 |
| 1874 | William Stevenson | 5,000 00 |

## T.

| | | | |
|---|---|---:|---:|
| 1772 | Peter Turner | $266 | 66 |
| 1774 | Thomas Turner | 400 | 00 |
| 1800 | William Topliff, merchant | 266 | 66 |
| 1810 | Thomas Topliff | 237 | 33 |
| 1818 | Margaret Thomas | 133 | 33 |
| 1819 | Dinah Thomas | 20 | 00 |

## V.

| | | | |
|---|---|---:|---:|
| 1870 | Eliza H. Vaux | 1,000 | 00 |

## W.

| | | | |
|---|---|---:|---:|
| 1754 | Edward Warner £25 0s. 0d. | | |
| 1768 | Edward Warner's heirs; viz., Joseph Fox, Mary and Sarah Norris, Anna Warner, Joshua Howell, and Sam'l Shoemaker, present a residuary balance of 103 5 10 | 342 | 10 |
| 1763 | Abraham Waggoner | 53 | 33 |
| 1765 | Christopher Wilt | 160 | 00 |
| 1767 | Stephen Williams | 80 | 00 |
| " | Robert Wilson | 26 | 67 |
| 1772 | William White | 213 | 33 |
| 1773 | William Wood | 26 | 67 |
| 1783 | John Wall, of New Jersey | 933 | 39 |
| 1797 | Bartholomew Wistar | 266 | 66 |
| 1802 | William Wister | 133 | 33 |
| 1804 | William Wharton, ground rents of $39 50 per annum, at par | 658 | 33 |
| 1805 | Peter Wickoff | 100 | 00 |
| 1815 | Chamless Wharton | 500 | 00 |
| 1828 | John G. Wachsmuth | 1,950 | 00 |
| 1872 | R. D. Wood | 200 | 00 |

## Z.

| | | | |
|---|---|---:|---:|
| 1758 | Lloyd Zachary £350 0 0 | 1,112 | 12 |
| 1768 | "  his Exrs. and Devisees 67 11 0 | | |
| 1793 | Jonathan Zane (received from 1793 to 1800) | 889 | 15 |

## IX.

## DONATIONS.

#### FROM CORPORATIONS, ETC.

| Year | Donor | | | | Amount | Total |
|---|---|---|---|---|---|---|
| 1751 | Thornbury Township | | | | | $26 67 |
| 1762 | Middletown Township, Chester Co. | | | | | 150 66 |
| 1758 | Union Fire Company | £25 | 0s. | 0d. | | |
| 1763 | " | 10 | 0 | | | 81 33 |
| 1789 | " | 5 | 0 | 0 | | |
| 1759 | Friendship Fire Co. | | | | | 26 67 |
| 1786 | Concert in German Reformed Church | | | | | 110 95 |
| 1864 | First National Bank | | | | | 500 00 |
| " | Philadelphia Bank | | | | | 1,000 00 |
| " | City National Bank | | | | | 100 00 |
| " | Penn National Bank | | | | | 100 00 |
| 1858 | Saint Peter's Church | | | | | 100 00 |
| 1864 | The Phœnix Iron Co. | | | | | 250 00 |
| 1852 | The Philada. and Reading R. R. Co. | | | | 2,000 | |
| 1864 | " " " | | | | 10,000 | |
| 1867 | " " " | | | | 1,000 | |
| 1868 | " " " | | | | 1,000 | |
| 1869 | " " " | | | | 1,000 | |
| 1870 | " " " | | | | 1,000 | |
| 1871 | " " " | | | | 1,000 | 17,000 00 |
| 1864 | The Pennsylvania R. R. Co. | | | | 10,000 | |
| 1867 | " " | | | | 5,000 | 15,000 00 |
| 1864 | The Phila. W. & B. R. R. Co. | | | | 600 | |
| 1866 | " " " " | | | | 600 | |
| 1867 | " " " " | | | | 1,000 | |
| 1868 | " " " " | | | | 1,000 | |
| 1869 | " " " " | | | | 1,000 | |
| 1870 | " " " " | | | | 1,000 | |
| 1871 | " " " " | | | | 1,000 | 6,200 00 |
| 1864 | Lehigh Valley R. R. Co. | | | | 1,000 | |
| 1867 | " " " | | | | 300 | |
| 1868 | " " " | | | | 300 | |
| 1869 | " " " | | | | 300 | |
| 1870 | " " " | | | | 300 | |
| 1871 | " " " | | | | 300 | 2,500 00 |
| 1857 | Harrisburg, Lancaster & Portsmouth R. R. Co. | | | | | 500 00 |

| | | | | |
|---|---|---|---:|---:|
| 1867 | Schuylkill Navigation Co. | | | $300 00 |
| 1865 | Sanitary Commission | | $1,000 | |
| 1869 | " " | | 2,000 | 3,000 00 |

### Insurance Companies.

| | | | | |
|---|---|---|---:|---:|
| 1864 | Mutual Assurance | | 1,000 | |
| 1868 | " " | | 5,000 | 6,000 00 |
| 1864 | Insurance Co. of North America | | | 1,000 00 |
| " | Delaware Mutual Safety | | | 1,000 00 |
| " | Reliance Fire Co. | | | 200 00 |
| " | Mutual Life | | | 500 00 |
| 1867 | Philadelphia Contributionship Co. | | | 5,000 00 |

### From Individuals and Firms.

| | |
|---|---:|
| Charles Bartles, lumber | 50 00 |
| Cornelius Smith, in stock | 100 00 |
| James P. Wood, deduction from bill low steam apparatus | 100 00 |
| Rommel, Potts & Co., deduction from coal bill | 119 90 |
| George Dodd & Son, carriage work | 100 00 |
| Supplee & Pennepacker, deducted from bill, plastering | 250 00 |
| John G. Reading, lumber | 50 00 |
| Baker, Davis & Co., deducted from bill of books | 53 00 |
| Wm. D. Rodgers, deduction in price of pony phaeton | 65 00 |
| George Vogt, deduction in price of piano | 200 00 |

## X.

## CONTRIBUTORS TO THE PENNSYLVANIA HOSPITAL, 1751 TO 1876.

### A.

1751 William Allen, Esq., Ch'f Justice.
" Stephen Anthony.
" John Armitt, cooper.
1754 William Attwood.
" Alexander Allair.
" George Asbridge.
" Matthias Aspden.
1755 Benjamin Armitage, Jr., smith.
1759 Captain Henry Ash, mariner.
1761 Martin Ashburn.
" Joshua Ash, Darby, Chester Co.
1764 William Ashbridge, miller, Oxford Township.
1767 Lawrence Anderson.
1775 Joseph Allen.
1781 Chamless Allen.
1785 Richard Adams.
1786 Joseph Anthony, merchant.
" Peter Aston.
" John Angres.
1788 Thomas Affleck (in furniture).
1791 James Ash, Esq., sheriff.
" Thomas Powell Anthony.
1801 Robert Annesley, merchant.
1806 Robert Adams, merchant.
1809 John Ashley.
1821 William Abbott, brewer.
1832 Robert Andrews.
1833 Thomas Astley.
" William V. Anderson, grocer.
1841 Richard Ashhurst, merchant.
" Lewis R. Ashhurst, merchant.
1845 Joseph B. Andrews, lumber merchant.
" William Ashbridge.
1847 John Ashhurst.
" William L. Ashhurst.
1856 Richard Ashhurst, Jr.
" Joseph Andrade.
" S. Austin Allibone.
" Anthony J. Antelo.
" Ellis S. Archer.
1856 Mary Ann Archer.
" Jacob T. Alberger & Co.
" John Anspach.
" Joshua W. Ash.
" John Agnew.
" John B. Austin.
" Jacob Alter.
" Geo. R. Ayres.
" George Abeel.
1857 Abbott & Lawrence.
" Thomas Allibone.
" William L. Abbott.
1858 James Andrews.
" Lewis Audenreid.
1859 John C. Allen.
" Samuel Ashhurst.
" John Ashhurst, Jr.
" Jane Ashbridge.
" Thomasin Ashbridge.
" Allen & Needles.
1860 Mrs. Lewis R. Ashhurst.
" Andrews & Dixon.
" W. & J. Allen.
1865 D. Hayes Agnew, M.D.
1867 William H. Ashhurst.
1868 Dr. Francis Ashhurst.
1873 W. Ashmead, M.D.

### B.

1751 Anthony Benezet.
" John Bleakley, shopkeeper.
" Dr. Thomas Bond.
" Dr. Phineas Bond.
1752 Daniel Benezet.
" John Bowman.
" William Branson, merchant.
" John Bayley.
" William Ball, goldsmith.
" William Bard, merchant.
" John Baynton.
1754 Gunning Bedford, carpenter.
" Philip Benezet, merchant.

1754 John Biddle.
" Samuel Bonnel, smith.
" Thomas Bourne.
" Thomas Brooks, bricklayer.
" Jeremiah Brown.
" George Bullock.
" John Bringhurst, merchant.
1755 William Bradford.
" John Bleakley, Sr.
" Andrew Bankson.
" William Buckley.
1756 Henry Bossler, innkeeper.
" George Bensell.
" Samuel Burge.
" James Benezet.
" George Bryan.
1758 John and Jacob Bankson.
" John Bissell, smith.
" Joseph Baker.
" William Bingham, Sr.
1759 John Bell
" Richard Blackham.
1761 David Bacon, hatter.
" James Bringhurst, house carpenter.
" Joseph Bringhurst, cooper.
" Matthias Bush.
" John Baily (furniture).
1762 David Barclay and Sons, London.
" Davis Bassest.
1763 Job Bacon, hatter.
" Abraham Bickley, merchant.
1764 David Beveridge, merchant.
1766 Captain Richard Budden.
" Elias Bland (fire engine).
" Timothy Bevan, London.
1767 Clement Biddle, merchant.
1768 Robert Bass.
" John Bayard, merchant.
1769 John Bringhurst, of Germant'n.
1770 William Barrell.
1771 James Biddle, Esq.
" George Bertram.
1773 Morris Birkbeck, of Gt. Britain.
1775 Barnabas Barnes.
" Edward Bonsall.
1780 Hillary Baker.
1781 William Bingham.
1786 Peter Baynton.
" Jacob Biker.
" Edward Bird.
" John Bartholomew.
" William Bradford, Jr.
" Captain Thomas Bell.
" Robert Bridges.
" J. J. Burchell.
" Joseph Blewer.
" Daniel Byrnes.
1787 Edward Brooks.
1788 Cornelius Barnes.
1793 Robert Buchanan, of Scotland.
1794 David Breintnall.
" Frederick Boller.
1795 Samuel Baker, hatter.
1797 Paul Beck, Jr., merchant.
" Peter Brown.
" Samuel Blodget.
1798 Dr. Benjamin S. Barton.
1799 Joseph Ball, merchant.
" Andrew Brown, printer.
1801 Robert Barclay, merchant.
1802 George Branner, milkman.
" Anthony M. Buckley, merchant.
" Samuel Brown.
1803 John Bacon, merchant.
1804 Jacob Beninghove, tobacconist.
1807 Thomas Biddle, broker.
" John Coates Brown, shipsmith.
" William J. Brown.
" Curtis Bolton, merchant.
1809 John Bolton, of Savannah.
" Matthew L. Bevan, merchant.
1810 Horace Binney, Esq., attorney-at-law.
1812 Joshua Byron.
1818 John R. Baker.
1820 Charles Bird.
1821 Joseph D. Brown.
1823 John Rhea Barton, M.D.
1824 Josiah Bunting, lumber merch't.
1827 John Bell, M.D.
" Franklin Bache, M.D.
1828 Edward Burd.
1833 Theophilus E. Beesley, M.D.
1834 David S. Brown, merchant.
" Jeremiah Brown, merchant.
" William Henry Brown, merchant.
1840 Frederick Brown, apothecary.
1841 James H. Bradford, M.D.
1815 Clement C. Biddle.
1846 John B. Biddle, M.D.
1847 Issac Barton.
1848 Jacob T. Bunting.
1849 William Biddle.
" T. Hewson Bache, M.D.
1851 Samuel Bettle, Jr.
" William Bettle.
1852 Charles L. Boker.
" Henry Paul Beck.
" Geo. W. Biddle.
" Charles S. Boker, M.D.
" Ann M. Biker.
" Charles H. Baker.
" Frederick Brown, Jr.
1853 Washington Brown.
1854 Clement Biddle, Jr.
" Thomas A. Biddle.
1855 Henry I. Biddle.
" Bennerville D. Brown.
" Alexander Biddle.

1855 James Bayard.
" Jona. Williams Biddle.
1856 M. Brook Buckley.
" Timothy M. Bryan.
" Abraham Barker.
" Albert Barnes.
" Charles Borie.
" Joseph B. Bloodgood.
" W. G. Boyd.
" John Bohlen.
" John A. Brown.
" William A. Blanchard.
" John B. Budd.
" Samuel Branson.
" Thomas Beaver.
" Bucknor, McCammon & Co.
" Maria Blight.
" Moses Brown.
" William H. Brown & Co.
" Alexander Brown.
" Joel J. Baily.
" Pierre Antoine Blenon.
" Thomas Biddle.
1857 H. Nelson Burroughs.
" Brown & Embly.
" John M. Butler.
" Henry P. Borie.
" William M. Baird.
" Patrick Brady.
" James Benners.
" Stephen Baldwin.
" Budd & Comley.
" Bates & Coats.
" E. F. Bockius.
" Bute & Smith.
" Samuel Barton & Co.
" William Bucknall.
" William E. Bowen.
" Washington Butcher.
" John Butcher.
" Alexander Benson.
" Gustavus S. Benson.
" Matthew W. Baldwin & Co.
" Stacey B. Barcroft.
" Bunn, Raiguel & Co.
" Horace Binney, Jr.
" John W. Biddle.
" Samuel Biddle.
" Boulton, Vandevere & Co.
" George H. Burgess, M.D.
" S. S. Brown.
" H. S. Benson.
" John Bohlen, Jr.
1858 Bailey & Brothers.
" Mary Bray.
" M. & C. Bancroft.
" Josiah Bacon.
" John A. Brown (builder).
" Joseph M. Bennett.
1859 Atherton Blight.
" T. W. & M. Brown.

1859 John Baird.
" Michal & Baker.
" Joshua L. Bailey.
" Edward Bedlock.
" John P. Brock.
" John C. Bullitt.
" Robert Buist.
" Elizabeth C. Biddle.
" Benjamin Bullock.
" Dr. James Bond.
" Henry M. Benners.
" George W. Benners.
" Samuel Branson,
" Jane Brinton.
" George Brinton.
" Samuel Baugh.
" Allen H. Bookhammer.
" Joseph Budd.
" Lewis Brinton.
" Andrew C. Barclay.
" Dr. George H. Burgin.
" T. Wistar Brown.
" William S. Baird.
1860 Henry B. Benners.
" Mrs. Moses Brown.
" Mrs. A. E. Borie.
" Mrs. Ball.
" Mrs. Horace Binney.
" Mrs. Christian Biddle.
" Mrs. John B. Budd.
" Mrs. John A. Brown.
" William Brown.
" Clement B. Barclay.
" John Brock.
" John Black.
" Charles Bullock.
" William S. Boyd.
1861 Michael Bouvier.
1864 Mary D. Brown.
" Emily M. Biddle.
" Clement Biddle.
" Adolph E. Borie.
" J. H. Bracken.
" William H. Boyer.
1865 Helen Bell.
" S. Mason Bines.
" S. Mason Bines, Jr.
" William T. Bines.
" David A. Bines.
" Bowen & Fox.
" Jairus Baker.
" Emily Bell.
" Ann M. Baker.
1866 Boyd & Hough.
" Richard W. Bacon.
" Andrew C. Barclay.
" Charles P. Bayard.
1867 Laura Bell.
" C. & H. Borie.
" John R. Blackiston.

1867 Joseph Bacon.
" Robert & W. E. Biddle.
" E W. Bailey.
" Theodore Bliss.
" Henry Bower.
" Mrs. Wm. Bucknell.
" Alfred G. Baker.
" Matthew Baird.
" Edward S. Buckley.
" B. H. Bartol.
" John Boulton.
" Bement & Dougherty.
" Mrs Thomas A. Biddle.
" Francis Blackburne, Jr.
" Mrs. Frederick Brown, Sr.
" Charlotte Aug'a Brown.
1870 Mary S Brown.
1871 Mark Balderston.
" Thomas A. Boyd.
1872 Sydney A. Biddle.
" Arthur Biddle.
1874 T. Hewson Bradford, M.D.
1875 Mrs. Wm. A. Blanchard.
" Maria E. Blanchard.
1876 Isabella Brown.
" Alexander P. Brown.
" Clement M. Brown.

C.

1751 Thomas Cadwalader, M.D.
" Joshua Crosby, gentleman.
1752 Thomas Crosby.
1754 Samuel Caruthers, joiner.
" William Chancellor, M D.
" James Chattin, printer.
" James Child, merchant.
" John Church, of Wicaco.
" William Campfler, merchant.
" James Clulo, potter.
" Thomas Clifford, merchant.
" William Coleman, merchant.
" Jacob Cooper.
" John Cresson, whitesmith.
" Matthias Culp, innkeeper.
" William Cooper.
1755 John Coates.
" David Chambers, stonecutter.
" John Coates, Jr., brickmaker.
" Thomas Coates, Jr., brickmaker.
" James Coultas, mariner.
" Corncord Township (Chester Co.)
1756 Samuel Cheesman, shoemaker.
" Matthew Clarkson.
" Benjamin Chew, Esq.
" Thomas Carpenter.
" Redmond Conyngham.
1757 Jonathan Cowpland, mariner.
1758 Charles Coxe.

1758 Samuel Chancellor.
1759 William Clifton, smith.
" Peter Chevallier.
1761 John Correy.
" George Clymer, merchant.
" James Chalmers, of Jamaica.
" Emanuel Carpenter, of Lancaster Co.
" Daniel Clark.
" John Coxe, M.D.
" Isaac Coxe.
" William Coxe, Esq.
1762 Stephen Collins.
1763 James Cresson, carpenter.
1764 William Craig.
1765 Thomas Clifford.
1766 David Hayfield Conyngham.
1771 John Cadwalader.
" Samuel Coates.
1772 Joshua Cresson, merchant.
" Thomas Combe.
1773 Thomas Corbyn, John Brown, and John Beaumont, of London, in medicine.
1775 Joseph Crukshank, printer.
1776 Isaac Coates.
1780 John Clark.
" Tench Coxe.
1782 Joseph Copperthwaite.
1785 Josiah Coates.
1786 William Cox, chairmaker.
" William Coxe, Jr., merchant.
" John Chaloner.
" Samuel Caldwell.
" Curtis Clay.
1787 Samuel Clark.
1788 James Colbreath.
" Andrew Caldwell.
1794 Samuel Coates, Jr.
" John Reynell Coates.
1795 Zaccheus Collins, merchant.
1797 Joseph S. Coates.
1798 Josiah L. Coates.
" Samuel Cooper, M.D.
" Charles Caldwell, M.D.
" John Redmond Coxe, M.D.
1799 Rachael Crukshank.
1800 James Crukshank, bookseller.
1801 Alexander Cook, soap-boiler.
" William Chancellor.
1803 James W. Clement, merchant.
1806 Eli Canby, merchant.
" Andrew Caldcleugh, merchant of N. C.
" Lewis Clapier, merchant.
1807 Thomas Clayton, hatter.
" Nathaniel Chapman, M D.
" Charles Chauncy, attorney-at-law.
1809 Thomas P. Cope, merchant.

1810 Samuel Calhoun, M.D.
1813 Jasper Cope, merchant.
" George M. Coates, seedman.
" Thomas Cadwalader.
1815 Turner Camac.
" Sarah Camac.
1817 Israel Cope, merchant.
" Caleb Cresson.
1819 Richard P. Cummings, coppersmith.
" John Coulter, merchant.
1820 Benjamin Horner Coates, M D.
1822 John Cooke, merchant.
1826 J. Y. Clarke, M D.
1831 Robert A. Caldcleugh.
1833 Caleb Cope, merchant.
1838 Thomas F. Cock, M.D.
1840 Allen Clapp, steward Pennsylvania Hospital.
" Andrew D. Cash, conveyancer.
1845 Daniel W. Coxe.
" Edward Coles.
" John Curwen, M.D.
1847 Elliott Cresson.
" William Chancellor.
1848 Robert Coleman.
1849 Joseph Carson, M.D.
" Henry Cramond.
1851 Charles Conrad.
1852 Jane Clark.
" John Conrad.
" William Camac, M.D.
" Solomon Conrad.
" John Canby.
1854 Charles S. Coxe.
" Brinton Coxe.
" Alexander B. Coxe.
" Ecley B. Coxe.
" Henry B. Coxe.
" Charles B. Coxe.
1855 Nathaniel Chauncey.
" John P. Crozier.
" Wharton Chancellor.
1856 Martin Curren.
" George Cadwalader.
" George C. Carson.
" Cochran & Russell.
" Alfred Cope.
" Samuel J. Christian.
" Harriet Coleman.
" Francis R. Cope.
" Thomas P. Cope.
" William Cummings.
" Henry Cope.
" Aaron B. Cooley.
" Coffin Colket.
" John E. Cope.
" Andrew R. Chambers.
" Henry Croskey.
" Caldwell & English.

1856 James L. Claghorn.
" Andrew C. Craig.
" Arthur G. Coffin.
" John C. Cresson.
" Enoch W. Clark.
" Wm. C. Coats.
" S. Wilmer Connell.
" T. K. & P. G. Collins.
" Henry C. Carey.
" William Clark.
" Julius K. Clark.
1857 Joseph Cresson.
" Hugh Campbell.
" Cabeen & Co.
" Jay Cooke.
" Jas. R. Campbell.
" Hagan Carney.
" John Cadwallader.
" Daniel B. Cummings.
" B. B. Comegys.
" Frederick Collins.
" John Cox.
" Wm. Carpenter.
" Francis Carpenter.
" Alexander G. Cattell.
" James Cresson.
" Benjamin T. Curtis.
" Joseph H. Campion.
" Henry Croskey & Co.
" Abraham Coates.
" Charles C. Cresson.
" M. H. Cobb.
" Sarah T. Curtis.
" Wm. B. Cazenove.
1858 Churchman, Craig & Co.
" Allen Cuthbert.
" Franklin A. Comly.
" J. K. Collins.
" Samuel Castner.
" Joseph H. Collins.
" James W. Claghorn.
" George Cromelien.
" Joseph R. Chandler.
" H. H. Catherwood.
" Hannah W. Collins.
" Wm. P. Cresson.
" Charles H. Cummings.
" Charles Camblos.
" Edward W. Clark.
1859 Benjamin Coates.
" Stephen Colwell.
" Mrs. D. M. Chambers.
" Daniel Corbit.
" Robert Creighton.
" Carter & Scattergood.
" John Clark.
" Eliza G. Cattell.
" Abigail Cooper.
" Edward S. Coxo.
" G. Dawson Coleman.

1859 William J. Caner.
" Childs & Peterson.
" Carwen Stoddart & Bro.
" Charles H. Clark.
" John Carter.
" James E. Caldwell & Co.
" Miss H. Cooper.
" Mrs. Crozier.
1860 Ephraim Clark, Jr.
" Cornelius & Baker.
" Prudent Castamajor.
" Archibald Campbell.
" John E Carter.
" Theo. Cuyler.
" D. B. Cummings.
" Mrs. J. W. Cannell.
1864 Charles W. Churchman.
" E. W. Clark & Co.
" Coffin & Altemus.
" Cabeen & Co.
" Emlen Cresson.
" A. W. Cummings.
" Geo. W. Childs.
1865 Esther L. Cooper.
" James M. Crossman.
" Thomas Craven.
" Samuel F. Canby.
1866 Hamilton Creighton. Esq.
" Robert Coburn.
1867 Jay Cooke & Co
" Franklin A. Comley, Jr.
" Cain, Hacker & Cook.
" Wm. D. Cope.
" James S. Cox.
" Elias Cope.
" Hetty L. Cooper.
1868 Clarence H. Clark.
1869 George R. Creely
1870 George M. Conarroe.
" Edwin R. Cope.
1871 M. J. Coleman.
" Jerome Carter.
1874 St. Geo. T. Campbell.

D.

1752 David Deshler.
1754 William Dowell.
" Daniel Dupuy, silversmith.
" Andrew Doz.
" Thomas Davis, merchant.
" Jacob Duchee, Esq.
" Edward Duffield, watchmaker.
1756 William Dilworth, carpenter.
" John Drinker, bricklayer.
1757 David Davis (in lumber).
1758 Matthew Drason.
1759 Robert Dixon, innkeeper.
" Henry Drinker.

1759 William Denny.
1761 Charles Dingee.
1763 George Dillwyn, merchant.
1764 John Dickenson, Esq.
1765 William Dickenson.
1771 Sharpe Delany, druggist.
" Daniel Drinker, merchant.
" Samuel Duffield, M.D.
1772 Benedict Dorsey, grocer.
1773 Joseph Dean.
1782 Henry Diering, of Lancaster.
1785 Leonard Dorsey.
" William Dawson.
1786 John Donnaldson.
" William Delany.
1787 John David, silversmith.
1793 John Dorsey.
1794 Andrew Douglas.
1795 Jonathan Dawes.
" John Dunlap, printer.
1796 Abijah Dawes.
1798 Robert Dawson, merchant.
1801 William Dillwyn, of Great Britain.
1805 William P. Dewees, M.D.
1807 Florimond Dusar, merchant.
" John Syng Dorsey, M.D.
1808 Samuel F. Dawes, merchant.
1809 John Dayton.
1813 Jacob Downing.
1815 David Jones Davis, M.D.
1816 Bernard Dahlgren.
1827 Isaac Davis, tanner.
1832 Nathan Dunn, merchant.
" Mordecai L. Dawson, brewer.
1844 William H. Dillingham, attorney-at-law.
1849 James Dundas.
1852 William M. Dawson.
" Joseph Dingee.
1855 Alexander J. Derbyshire.
1856 Benj. J. Douglas.
" Joseph H. Dallas.
" Dallett Brothers.
" Dawson & Hancock.
" Isaac R. Davis.
" Levi Dickson.
" James N. Dickson.
" Sally N. Dickinson.
" Josiah Dawson.
" Benj. Davis.
" Ellwood Davis.
1857 Gillies Dallett.
" Henry Duhring.
" Sophia Donaldson.
" Elijah Dallett.
" John Devereux.
" Mrs. Richard C. Dale.
" Charles Dutilth.
" Ferdinand J. Dreer.
" Michael Day.

1857 James C. Donnell.
" William A. Drown.
1858 John C. Davis.
" Dr. James C. Darrach.
1859 J. Perot Downing.
" Haward W. Drayton.
" John A. Dougherty.
" Charles A. Dougherty.
" William H. Dougherty.
" William Divine.
" Elizabeth Dawson.
" Edward M. Davis, Jr.
" William Dillworth.
" Stanton Dorsey.
" William Dorsey.
" Danforth, Wright & Co.
" Mrs. Joseph H. Dulles.
" H. T. Desilver.
" Wm. Heyward Drayton.
1860 Thomas Drake.
" Miss M. Dixon.
" Miss S. Dixon.
" Mrs. R. C. Dale.
" Charles Desilver.
" Mrs. John Dallett.
" Wm. Dunlap.
1864 John Dobson.
" Mary A. Derbyshire.
1865 Anthony J. Drexel.
" Smedley Darlington.
" De Haven & Brother.
" J. M. DaCosta, M.D.
1867 Henry Disston.
" Drexel & Co.
" J. Russell Dawson.
1868 Henry K. Dillard.
" Wm. A. Drown, Jr.
1872 Moses A. Dropsie.

E.

1754 George Emlen, Sr., brewer.
" Samuel Emlen.
" Jeremiah Elfreth.
" Thomas Ellis, glazier.
" Edward Evans, shoemaker.
1755 Joshua Emlen.
1756 Jonathan Evans.
1758 Robert Erwin.
" James Eddy.
1761 Andrew Elliott.
1766 Thomas Eastburn.
1771 John Evans, hatter.
1773 Joel Evans.
1781 George Emlen, Jr.
1785 Thomas Ewing.
" Paul Engle.
1786 George Eddy.
1787 Thomas Eddy.

1787 John Elliott, druggist.
1796 John Elliott, Jr., druggist.
1798 Samuel Elam, merchant of R. I.
" Robert Elam, merchant of G. B.
" Gervas Elam, merchant of G. B.
1800 Josiah Evans, plasterer.
" Edward Evans, plasterer.
1802 Nathan Eyre, tailor.
1803 Hugh Ely, merchant.
1806 Joseph Bennett Eves, merchant.
" Jonathan Evans, lumber merchant.
1807 Charles C. Evans, carpenter.
1809 Alexander Elmslie, merchant.
1810 Ann K. Eyre.
1813 Maria K. Eyre.
1822 Samuel Emlen, M.D.
1826 Governeur Emerson, M.D.
1833 Isaac Elliott, conveyancer.
" Charles Evans, M.D.
1840 Thomas Evans, apothecary.
1845 Charles Ellis, apothecary.
1847 Adam Eckfeldt.
1850 George M. Elkinton.
1852 William Ellis.
" Lindley M. Elton.
1855 Joshua P. Eyre.
1856 Thomas Estlack.
" Samuel W. Earl.
" John Eisenbray, Jr.
" Thomas Earp.
" Michael Errickson.
" Andrew M. Eastwick.
" John B. Ellison & Sons.
" Charles Ellis & Co.
" Edward Evans.
" John T. Epplesheimer.
1857 Joseph R. Evans.
" Rowland G. Evans.
" George W. Edwards.
" Robert Ewing.
" Thomas Earp, Jr.
" Evans & Watson.
1858 Horace Evans, M.D.
" John Evans.
1859 J. Livingston Erringer.
" Wm. Ebbs.
1860 Jane Evans.
" R. and M. Ely.
" William Evans, Jr.
" Mrs. John H. Irwin.
1864 John Eisenbery & Sons.
" J. Wistar Evans.
" Adam Everly.
1865 John Elliott.
" Lucy H. Eddy.
" William Elmsley.
" Rebecca Elmsley.
" Ann Elmsley.
" Elizabeth Elmsby.

1866 Thomas Earle.
1870 Charles Evans.
1873 Mary L. Erwin.
1875 John Embley.

### F.

1751 William Fishbourne.
" Joshua Fisher.
" Enoch Flowers.
" Joseph Fox.
" Benjamin Franklin, printer.
1752 Richard Farmer, M.D.
" Solomon Fussel, merchant.
1754 Hugh Forbes.
" William Franklin.
" William Fisher.
1755 Standish Ford, innkeeper.
" David Franks.
1756 Plunket Fleeson.
1758 Judah Foulke.
" Samuel Fisher.
" Lester Falkner.
1759 John Franks.
1764 Ferdinand Farmer.
" Robert Field.
1765 John Fothergill, M.D.
1768 Thomas Fisher.
" Captain Nathaniel Falconer.
1770 Caleb Foulke.
1771 Samuel Fisher, Jr.
1772 Thomas Forrest.
" William Fisher, Jr.
" John Field, merchant.
1775 Samuel Fisher, butter.
1776 Ludwig Falkenstine.
1782 William Forbes.
1784 John Foulke, M D.
1785 Miers Fisher.
1786 William Folwell.
" George Fox.
" Nalbro Frazer.
" Joseph Few.
1794 Samuel M. Fox, merchant.
1796 James C. Fisher, merchant.
1801 John Folwell, merchant.
" Samuel W. Fisher, merchant.
1802 Walter Franklin, attorney-at-law
1807 Thomas W. Francis, merchant.
1808 Redwood Fisher, merchant.
1811 Robert Fielding, coachmaker.
1819 Samuel Fox, brickmaker.
1824 William W. Fisher.
1826 Samuel M. Fox, M.D.
1829 William B. Fling.
1833 Stephen G. Fotterall.
1834 Alexander Fullerton, Jr., druggist.
1835 George Fox, M.D.

1844 Samuel T. Fisher.
1845 John Farnum, merchant.
" Mary P. Fisher.
1848 Frederick Fraley.
1852 Aaron Fogg.
" W. S. Forbes, M.D.
1855 Joseph Fisher.
" Alfred Fassett.
" Jason L. Fennimore.
1856 George W. Farnum.
" Bartholomew Wistar Fellows.
" Fearons & Smith.
" Charles Henry Fisher.
" John Fallon.
" Christopher Fallon.
" F. T. Fiqueira.
" Field & Keebmle.
" Fales, Lothrop & Co.
" David Faust.
" J. Gillingham Fell.
" Rodney Fisher.
" John C. Farr.
" Alexander Fullerton.
1857 Charles P. Fox.
" Franklin Fell.
" William B. Foster.
" George W. Fobes.
" Stephen Fuquet.
" B. A. Fahnestock.
" James Field.
" Henry Fling.
" William Fling (Mcht.).
" Mrs. William Fling.
" J. Francis Fisher.
" Mary P. Fisher.
" George W. Farnum.
1858 Field & Hardie.
" John M. Ford.
" Furness, Brinley & Co.
" Charles S. Folwell.
1859 H. N. Fitzgerald.
" B. B. Fahnestock & Co.
" Frederick Fairthorn.
" French, Richards & Co.
" Jacob Freas.
" A. J. Flomerfelt.
" Fithian, Jones & Co.
" Eliza G. Fisher.
" Ellen Fisher.
1860 William B. Foster, Jr.
" Mrs. G. W. Fahnestock.
" Thomas Firth.
" Miss Mary Fox.
" Wm. H. French.
" Mrs. and Miss W. W. Fisher.
" Elizabeth H. Farnum.
" Susan Farnum.
" Mary Farnum.
1864 Frothingham & Wells.
1865 Charles A. Farnham.

1865 Rebecca Ann Fell.
" Fricken & Williams.
1867 George Fales.
" Samuel M. Fox.
" John Fagan.
" Fitler, Weaver & Co.
" Fara & Brothers.
" S. & J. M. Flanagan.
" John W. Forney.
" Charles J. Fields.
1876 Eliza Freeman.

G.

1751 Thomas Græme, M.D.
" Isaac Greenleafe.
" William Griffiths.
1754 George Gray, brewer.
" William Grant.
" Joseph Galloway.
" Isaac Garrigues.
" Joseph Gibbons.
" Walter Goodman.
" Thomas Gordon.
" Christian Grassheld, tailor.
" Joseph Greenway.
1755 Joseph Gray.
" Nathaniel Grubb.
" David George.
" Joseph Gamble, of Barbadoes.
" George Gray, Jr., Lower Ferry.
1757 Sebastian Graff.
" John Goodwin, Jr.
1761 John Grandom, tailor.
" John Gibson.
1762 Lawrence Growdon, Esq.
" William Gibbons.
1763 Jacob Graff, bricklayer.
1865 Lord Adam Gordon.
" Andrew Henry Groth.
1769 William Gale, of Jamaica.
" Henry Hale Graham, of Chester Co.
1776 James Glenn.
1783 Samuel Garrigues, Jr.
1786 Stephen Girard.
1788 Samuel P. Griffitts, M.D.
1790 Benjamin Gibbs.
1795 Thomas Greeves, merchant.
1796 Francis Gurney, merchant.
" Josiah Willard Gibbs
" Thomas George, of Blockley.
" Edward Garrigues, carpenter.
1801 Peter Grellet, merchant
1806 Abraham M. Garrigues, merchant.
1807 William Gerhard, farrier.
1812 Thomas Gilpin.
" Joshua Gilpin.
1815 Simon Gratz, merchant.

1817 John R. Griffiths, slater.
1818 James R. Greeves, carpenter.
" Samuel Griscom.
1821 William Gibson, M.D.
1835 William W. Gerhard, M.D.
1836 Thomas George, iron merchant.
1842 Benjamin Gerhard, attorney-at-law.
1852 James Galliard.
" Thomas Greeves.
1853 George Gordon.
" Charles Gibbons.
1855 Henry Grove.
" Eliza P. Gurney.
" Robert E. Gray.
" Rebecca Gumbes.
1856 Grove & Brother.
" William E. Garrett.
" William Glading.
" William D. Gillespie.
" John Gibson.
" John Grigg.
" Samuel Grant, Jr.
" L. W. Glenn.
" Edward Garrett.
" Henry R. Gilbert.
1857 John Garrison.
" Greiner & Harkness.
" Jane Gibbons.
" Eliza Ann Graff.
" Gans, Leberman & Co.
" Isaac P. Garrett.
" John R. Gheen.
" Francis R. Gatchel.
" Jesse George.
1858 John Gilbert & Co.
" Henry D. Gilpin.
" William Gaul.
" John Gibson, Son & Co.
" T. L. Gillespie.
1859 G. W. Gorgas.
" David George.
" Abraham Gibbons.
" James Graham & Co.
" Eliza Gilpin.
" Rebecca George.
" William F. Griffiths.
" Edwin Greble.
" Elizabeth Greeves.
1860 Robert H. Gratz.
1865 V. & J. F. Gilpin.
" Rebecca Gratz.
1866 Mary Gilbert.
1867 Gaw, Bacon & Co.
" Walter Garrett.
" William E. Garrett, Jr.
" Louis A. Godey.
" Rebecca Gibson.
1870 E. B. Gardette.
" John F. Gilpin.

## H.

- 1751 David Hall.
- " Adam Harker.
- " Arent Hassert.
- " Joshua Howell.
- " John Hughes.
- 1752 Samuel Hazard, merchant.
- 1754 Edward Hicks.
- " Charles Harrison.
- " Michael Hillegas, merchant.
- " George Hitner, shopkeeper.
- " Enoch Hobart.
- " Thomas Holland, merchant.
- " Michael Holling, baker.
- " Samuel Howell, merchant.
- " William Hudson, farmer.
- 1755 John Hatkinson.
- " Hugh Hewes.
- 1756 William Hopkins.
- " Thomas Hallowell, bricklayer.
- " Joseph Hillborn, merchant.
- " Charles Humphreys.
- 1757 Joshua Humphreys (in lumber).
- " Eleanor Hair.
- 1758 John Head.
- " Samuel House, merchant.
- " Eden Haydock, plumber.
- " Josiah Hewes.
- 1759 James Hamilton, Governor.
- " Benjamin Hooton.
- " Robert Hamilton, of Manchester, Eng.
- " James Humphreys.
- " Henry Harrison.
- 1760 William Henderson.
- 1761 Andrew Hannis.
- " Roger Hunt, Esq.
- " Jonathan Harbine.
- 1762 John Hunt.
- " Adam Hoops.
- " Richard Hookley.
- " John Hannum, Esq.
- " Abraham Hendrick.
- " Reuben Haines, brewer.
- 1764 Benjamin Hammet, London.
- " Henry Hill.
- 1765 John Howard.
- " Amos Hillborn.
- " Samuel Hudson, merchant.
- 1766 George Halueker.
- 1768 William Hoffman, sugar-baker.
- " Isaac Howell, brewer.
- " Francis Hopkinson.
- " James Hunter, merchant.
- 1769 Benjamin Harbeson, coppersmith.
- " Jacob Harman.
- 1771 Adam Hubley.
- " Thomas Harpur.
- 1772 Samuel Howell, Jr.
- 1775 James Hartley.
- " William Hall.
- " Captain Robert Hardie.
- 1781 Israel Hallowell.
- " John Hood.
- 1782 John Hubley.
- 1783 Hugh Howell.
- " Robert Haydock.
- 1785 John Head, Jr.
- " Samuel Hodgdon.
- " Godfrey Haga, merchant.
- " Pattison Hartshorne, merchant.
- " Levi Hollingsworth.
- 1786 Caspar Wistar Haines.
- " John Hart.
- " Richard Hartshorne.
- 1787 George Hunter, M.D.
- " Isaac Hazlehurst.
- " Joseph Henszey.
- 1793 Jacob Hiltzheimer.
- 1795 Anna Head (Stewardson).
- 1796 Catharine Haines.
- " Isaac Harvey, Jr., merchant.
- 1797 Paschal Hollingsworth, merch't.
- 1798 Francis Higgins, Steward of P. H.
- 1800 James Hutton, ironmonger.
- 1801 Adam Herkness, stonecutter.
- " Thomas T. Hewson, M.D.
- 1803 Benjamin Horner, merchant.
- 1806 Henry Hollingsworth, merchant.
- " Reuben Haines.
- 1807 Joseph E. Howell.
- " Philip Whitfield Harvey, of Dublin, printer.
- 1810 Thomas Haskins, merchant.
- " Robert E. Hobart.
- 1811 Joseph Hartshorne, M.D.
- " Benjamin B. Howell.
- " Talbot Hamilton.
- 1812 Joseph P. Horner.
- 1821 Samuel Haydock, plumber.
- 1822 William L. Hodge, merchant.
- " Rowland Parry Heylin, M.D.
- 1827 Hugh L. Hodge, M.D.
- 1828 Erskine Hazard.
- " Joshua Haven.
- " Thomas Harris, M.D.
- 1829 Robert M. Huston, M.D.
- " George Harrison.
- 1831 William E. Horner, M.D.
- " George Handy, hardware merchant.
- 1834 Hugh F. Hollingshead.
- " James Hutchinson.
- " Richard Harlan, M.D.
- 1835 John Haseltine.
- 1836 Thomas Hutchinson.
- " John G. Hoskins.
- " William Harris, M.D.

1841 Joseph C. Harris, broker.
1843 Edward Hartshorne, M.D.
1845 Robert P. Harris, M.D.
" William Hembel.
" J. Pemberton Hutchinson.
" William E. Hacker, merchant.
" Isaiah Hacker, merchant.
" Jeremiah Hacker, merchant.
" William R. Hanson.
1846 A. Fullerton Hazard, druggist.
" John Hinkle, butcher.
1852 Wm. D. Hunt, M.D.
" John Harding, Jr.
1855 Wm. P. Hinds.
1856 Josiah L. Harvey.
" Henry Hartshorne, M.D.
" Heron & Martin.
" A. Douglass Hall, M.D.
" Hildeburne & Bros.
" Charles Humphries.
" James C. Hand.
" Arthur H. Howell.
" Joseph Howell.
" William H. Hart.
" Benj. P. Hutchinson.
" George L. Harrison.
" Edward M. Hopkins.
" Henry H. Houston.
" Daniel B. Hinman.
" Hoskins, Heiskell & Co.
" Aaron A. Hurley.
" Haywood, per Hawkins.
" Mary Hibbard.
" William Hay.
" Mrs. W. E. Hornor.
" Abraham Hart.
1857 Herman Haupt.
" Morris L. Hallowell & Co.
" Marshall Hill.
" Philip R. Howard.
" Ann Harris.
" G. Craig Heberton, M.D.
" S. K. Hoxie.
" Thomas P. Hoopes.
" Isaac T. Hacker.
" Samuel Huston.
" William S. Hansell.
" S. P. Hancock.
" William Howell.
" George Howell.
" John A. Howell.
" George Henderson.
" N. P. & S. W. Hacker.
" Robert Hansell.
" May Humphries.
" Alexander E Horn.
1858 Harbert & Davis.
" William C. Houston.
" James Harmer.
" Howard & Co.

1858 A. W. Harrison.
" W. J. Horstman.
" Lewis Hayward.
" Silas F. Herring.
" Joseph Harrison, Jr.
" W. S. Helmuth, M.D.
" George Helmuth.
1859 Addinell Hewson, M.D.
" Edward Hopper.
" Alfred M. Harkness.
" Curtis Hoopes.
" Christian J. Hoffman.
" Jules Hanel.
" Geo. W. Harris.
" Heilwan & Rank.
" John Hulme.
" Mrs. W. Helmuth.
" Charles H. Hutchinson.
" Margaret J. Handy.
" Dr. Jas. H. Hutchinson.
1860 William Hopper.
" Mrs. M. A. Hodgson.
" James Harper.
" Morris L. Hallowell.
" Mrs. Geo. L. Harrison.
1863 George R. Harmstead.
" Samuel Hutchinson.
1864 Spencer H. Hazard.
" Hoopes & Townsend.
" Joseph Howell & Co.
" T. C. Henry & Co.
1865 Daniel Hendrie.
" Morris Hacker.
" William Hacker.
" Paschall Hacker.
" J. Barclay Hacker.
" T. G. Hollingsworth, Ex'rs of.
" Henry Haines.
1866 Jane R. Haines.
" Anton Heppman.
1867 Hammitt & Neal.
" Hoyt & Brother.
" James C. Hand & Co.
" Margaretta Hutchinson.
" Emlen Hutchinson.
" William Harmer.
" Homer, Colladay & Co.
" Dr. Henry C. Hart.
" Marshall Henzey.
" Edwin Henderson.
" Julia Harvey.
" Barnabas Hammitt.
" Howell Brothers.
" James G. Hardie.
" Wm. P. & Geo. W. Hacker.
" Madame Hardy.
" Mrs. E. Hayward.
" Houston & Collins.
1868 J. Henry Hentz.
" W. H. Horstman & Sons.

1869 Ann Hertzog.
" Massey Huston.
" Alfred Hunt.
1870 Elizabeth M. Hacker.
" Hannah M. Hacker.
" George C. Harlan, M.D.
" H. Lenox Hodge, M.D.
1872 George W. Hammersley.
1873 James Hopkins.
1874 Chas. T. Hunter.
1876 Dr. William Barton Hopkins.

## I & J.

1751 Derrick Janson.
" Charles Jones.
" Abel James.
" Isaac Jones, Esq.
1752 Robert Jenney, LL.D., Minister of Christ Church.
" Matthew Johns, cooper.
1754 John Jones, shoemaker.
" Robert Jones, of Lower Merion.
" Joseph Johnson, tinman.
1755 Joseph James.
" Joseph Jackman, of Barbadoes.
1759 William Jones.
" Joseph Jones, of Plymouth.
" William Ibison.
1761 Captain Daniel Joy.
" Edward Jones, baker.
" Abraham Jadah.
1762 Jacob Jones, baker.
1765 Joseph Jacobs.
" John Jekyll.
1768 Jacob Joner, of Lancaster Co.
" Richard Jackson, Esq. of London.
1770 Isaac Jones, carpenter.
1773 Robert Strettel Jones.
1774 John James.
1775 Owen Jones, Jr., merchant.
1776 William Johnson.
1779 Matthew Irwin.
1784 Herbert Jones.
1785 Ezra Jones.
1786 Leonard Jacoby.
" Norris Jones.
1787 Dominick Joyce.
" David Jackson, M.D.
" Richard Jones.
1788 John Johnson, of Germantown.
1794 John Jorden, grocer.
1795 Jonathan Jones, merchant.
1801 Isaac H. Jackson, merchant.
1803 Thomas Jones, merchant.
" James Jones, farmer.
1807 Thomas C. James, M.D.
1809 Joseph Jones.

1813 Joseph Johnson, ship chandler.
1817 Joseph L. Ingles.
1819 Isaac C. Jones, merchant.
" Samuel T. Jones.
1820 George W. Jones, painter.
" Jonathan Jones, of Bordeaux.
1822 Alexander W. Johnston.
1826 Joseph R. Jenks, flour merchant.
1831 George M. Justice.
1841 William P. Johnston, M.D.
1844 Watson Jenks, flour merchant.
1846 John Jordan, Jr., grocer.
1847 Caleb Jones.
" Antoinette Jordan.
1848 David Jayne, M.D., druggist.
1852 Samuel Jeans.
1855 James R. Ingersol.
" Joshua T. Jeans.
" Robert S. Johnson.
" William D. Jones.
" Jno. O. James.
1856 Samuel W. Jones.
" Lawrence Johnson.
" John Jordon, Jr.
" Joseph Jones.
" Benjamin S. Janney, M.D.
" John H. Irwin.
" Jeans & Scattergood.
1857 Samuel N. Jones.
" Jauretche & Carstairs.
" Louis Iungerich.
" Joseph R. Ingersoll.
" George R. Justice.
" Thomas Jeans.
" Israel H. Johnson.
" Joseph Jenns.
" Lewis Jans.
" Jacob P. Jones.
1858 Andrew M. Jones.
" Alfred D. Jessup.
" Chas. C. Jackson.
" Thomas C. James.
" James, Jeffries & Co.
" James, Kent & Santee.
1859 Mrs. Joseph Jones.
" Mrs. A. D. Jessup.
" Frederick L. John.
" Ruth Johnson.
" Chalkley Jeffries.
" B. Muse Jones.
" Eben C. Jayne.
" David W. Jayne.
" Mrs. Samuel W. Jones.
1860 Charles M. Jackson.
" Mrs. B. Muse Jones.
1861 Samuel Johnson.
" Randolph & Jenks.
" Philip S. Justice.
" Isaac T. Jones.
1864 Jay Cooke & Co.

1864 Wm. P. Jenks.
1865 Samuel Jones.
" Mrs. Edward C. Iungerich.
" S. Harvey Jones.
" Eliza F. Johnson.
1866 Lewis C. Iungerich.
1867 Sidney G. Johns.
" Isaac C. Jones, Jr.
" John H. Irwin.
" Owen Jones.
1868 John W. Jordon.
1869 Napoleon A. Jennings.
1870 Ewing Jordon.
" Charles Ingersoll.
" Russell H. Johnson.

### K.

1751 Joseph King.
" Matthias Koplin.
1754 Peter Keen, merchant.
" Mahlon Kirkbride.
" Paulus Kripner, shopkeeper.
" Marcus Kuhl.
" Edward Kuhl.
" Matthias Kensil, inkeeper.
1755 John Kearsley, M.D.
" John Knowles (in lumber).
1756 Edmund Kearney.
1759 Benjamin Kendal.
1761 Henry Kepple, merchant.
" Philip Kinsey.
1762 George Kreeble.
1769 Reynold Keen, alderman.
1770 Adam Kuhn, M.D.
1786 John Kaighn.
" Peter Knight.
" Frederick Kuhl.
1798 George Krebs.
1801 Frederick Kisselman, merchant.
" Reay King, merchant.
1807 Elisha Kane, merchant.
1814 Edmund Kimber.
1818 Hartman Kuhn.
1821 John Kenworthy, painter.
1835 Thomas S. Kirkbride, M.D.
1841 Thomas Kimber, merchant.
1855 Hartman Kuhn.
" William C. Kent.
1856 Ed. C. Knight.
" Thomas Kimber, Jr.
" Frederick V. Krug.
" David Kirkpatrick.
" William Kirkham.
" Dennis Kelley.
" H. Kellogg & Sons.
1857 Edwin T. Kirpatrick.
" John Kirkbride.
" Rowland Kirpatrick.

1857 Robert Kelton.
" William Kirk.
" Isaac Koons.
1858 Charles Koons.
" Ann W. Kirkbride.
" Anne J. Kirkbride.
" Jos. John Kirkbride.
" Josiah Kisterbock.
" Reeve L. Knight.
1859 Kirkpatrick, De Haven & Co.
" Charles Kelly.
" Elizabeth Kirkbride.
" John Ketchum.
" Catharine Klingman.
" Ann M. Knight.
1864 Alfred J. Kay.
1866 Edwin Kirkpatrick.
1867 Wm. H. Kirpatrick.
" Adam A. Konigmacher.
" Lizzie B. Kirkbride.
" Charles M. King, M.D.

### L.

1751 Thomas Lightfoot.
" Thomas Lawrence, Jr.
" Joseph Leech.
" Jacob Lewis.
1752 Joseph Lownes.
" Benjamin Loxley, carpenter (in work).
1754 William Logan.
1755 John Luke, of Barbadoes.
1756 James Lownes.
" John Lynn.
" Philip Ludwell, of Virginia.
1757 Benjamin Lay.
1758 William Lightfoot.
1759 Jeptha Lewis, of Gwynedd.
" Samuel Lloyd, merchant.
1760 Samuel Lewis, carpenter.
1761 Thomas Livezey, Jr.
" John Lukens, Surveyor-General.
" Thomas Leech.
1763 John Lownes.
1764 Joseph Lancaster, joiner.
1765 William Lloyd.
1766 Christopher Ludwick, baker.
" Georgh Legh, Vicar of Halifax, G. B.
1770 Ellis Lewis.
1771 Captain Charles Lyon.
1775 Mordecai Lewis.
1780 George Logan, M.D.
1785 Thomas Lieper.
" George Ludlam.
1786 Abraham Liddon.
" Ebenezer Large.
" Nathaniel Lewis.

1786 William Lewis, merchant.
" William Lewis, attorney-at-law.
1787 Henry Land, M.D. (medicines).
1791 Robert Lewis.
1792 William Lucas.
1794 Joseph Lownes, silversmith.
" Seth Lucas.
1795 David Lewis, insurance broker.
1796 Moses Levy, attorney-at-law.
1799 Joseph S. Lewis.
1802 Reeve Lewis, merchant.
" David Lee.
1806 Mordecai Lewis, Jr., merchant.
" Samuel Neave Lewis, merchant.
1810 Joseph Lea.
1812 Hannah Lewis, Jr. (Paul).
" Mary Lewis (Moore).
1816 Mahlon Lawrence.
" Josiah H. Lownes.
1819 Joshua Lippincott, auctioneer.
1820 James Lyle.
1826 René La Roche, M.D.
1828 Lawrence Lewis.
1829 Charles Lukens, M.D.
1831 William Lynch, merchant.
1832 James Leslie, carpenter.
" Robert Looney, plumber.
" Isaac S. Lloyd, merchant.
1833 Mordecai D. Lewis, merchant.
1840 John T. Lewis, merchant.
1843 Saunders Lewis, attorney-at-law.
1844 George T. Lewis.
1845 Lyon J. Levy, silk merchant.
" J. Smith Lewis.
" Joseph S. Lewis.
1848 William R. Lejée.
" Robert M. Lewis.
1851 Lawrence Lewis, Jr.
" Robert M. Lewis, Jr.
" Francis W. Lewis, M.D.
" David Lapsley.
1852 Isaac Lea.
" Francis Albert Lewis.
" Daniel A. Langhorne, M.D.
" Robert M. Lewis.
1853 Samuel N. Lewis, Jr.
1854 James Dundas Lippincott.
1856 James J. Levick, M.D.
" Benj. I. Leedom.
" William W. Longstreth.
" Joseph S. Lovering.
" Ludwig, Kneedler & Co.
" P. L Laguerenne.
" William T. Lowber.
" Lindsay & Blackiston.
" Jacob B. Lancaster.
" Casper P. Lukens, M.D.
" Leaury & Sister.

1856 Charles S. Lewis.
" George Lewis.
1857 Edward Lowber.
" Martha R Lewis.
" Edwin M. Lewis.
" Abel Lincoln.
" Charles Leland.
" Anna M. Lewis.
" Edward E Law.
" George Lippincott.
" Joshua Longstreth.
" Joseph B. Lapsley.
" Maria D. Logan.
" Mary Anna Longstreth.
" Levick, Raisin & Co.
" Lightfoot & Walton.
1858 James M. Linnard.
" Henry C. Lea.
" Frederick Leibrandt.
" J. B. Lippincott & Co.
" R. F. Loper.
1859 Francis S. Lewis.
" John Lindsay.
" John Lambert.
" David Landreth.
" Lippincott & Parry.
" James Long.
" Sarah M. Livezey.
" Mrs. Edward Law.
1860 Miss Mary Lewis.
" Miss Elizabeth W. Lewis.
" Miss Sarah Lewis.
" Anna W. Lapsley.
" Frederick Lennig,
" F. Mortimer Lewis.
" Lewis Thompson & Co.
" Miss A. Lennig.
" Miss A. M. Lewis.
1863 Joseph Lea.
" David Oldham Lewis.
" Edward Livezey, M.D.
1864 Henry Lawrence.
" John T. Lewis & Bros.
" John Livezey.
" Henry Lewis.
1865 Mrs. Lawrence Lewis.
" William H. Larned.
" Elizabeth W. Lewis.
" J. Fisher Leaming.
1867 D. Landreth & Co.
" Charles Lennig.
" John B. Love.
" Thomas C. Love.
" William T. Leech.
" Charles E Lex.
1870 John T. Lewis, Jr.
1871 Dr. Richard J. Levis.
1873 Morris J. Lewis.
1875 David M. Lutz.

## M.

- 1751 Anthony Morris, brewer.
- " Anthony Morris, Jr.
- " Jonathan Mifflin, merchant.
- " Robert Moore.
- " George Mifflin.
- " Samuel Mifflin.
- " Wright Massey.
- " William Moode,
- " Evan Morgan,
- " Samuel Mifflin, of New Jersey.
- " Joseph Morris.
- " Rees Meredith.
- " John Mifflin.
- 1752 Samuel Preston Moore.
- " John Mease.
- 1754 William Masters.
- " William Moore.
- " Thomas Maddox.
- " Joshua Morris, of Abington.
- " Christopher Marshall.
- " Hugh Matthews.
- " Leonard Melchior, shopkeeper.
- " Charles Meredith.
- " Benjamin Mifflin.
- " John Mifflin, Jr.
- " George Miller.
- " Charles Moore, hatter.
- " James Murgatroyd, merchant.
- " Jacob Mang.
- " Samuel Morris, Sheriff.
- " Joseph Marriot.
- 1755 Thomas Maule.
- " Joseph Mather, miller.
- 1756 Luke Morris.
- " William Morris, Jr.
- " Thomas Moore.
- 1757 John Morris (lime).
- 1758 John McMichael.
- " Samuel Morris, Jr.
- " John Malcolm, sailmaker.
- " Samuel Massey.
- 1759 Benjamin Morgan.
- 1760 John Moland, Jr.
- 1761 Captain William Morrell.
- " Allen McLane, leather-dresser.
- " Samuel Morton, merchant.
- " Samuel McCall.
- " Edward Milner.
- " Abraham Mason, tailor.
- " Charles Moore, M.D.
- " John McPherson.
- " Robert Morris, merchant.
- 1762 Mildred and Roberts, London.
- " McLean and Stewart.
- 1764 John Morton, merchant.
- " Peter Miller conveyancer.
- " Esther Mifflin.
- " Edward Milner, miller.
- 1765 Thomas Mayberry.
- " John Mease, Jr.
- " Cadwalader Morris.
- " John Morgan.
- " Archibald McCall.
- 1767 Thomas Mifflin.
- 1768 James McCracken.
- 1773 Levi Marks.
- 1775 Thomas Marriot, farmer.
- " Samuel Miles.
- " Benjamin Marshall.
- " Joseph Mifflin.
- 1780 Thomas Morris, brewer.
- 1781 Blair McClenachan, merchant.
- " Robert Morton.
- 1784 John F. Mifflin.
- 1785 Jonathan Mifflin.
- 1786 James Miller.
- " Magnus Miller.
- " John Marshall.
- " Thomas Murgatroyd.
- " William McMurtrie.
- " Samuel Meredith.
- 1787 John McCulloch.
- " James McCrea.
- " Benjamin Wistar Morris.
- " Patrick Moore.
- 1788 Christain Marshall, Jr.
- " Charles Marshall.
- 1796 John Morris, M.D.
- 1800 Richard Hill Morris
- 1801 Israel Maul, carpenter.
- " Thomas Morris, Jr., brewer.
- " Joseph S. Morris, brewer.
- " Charles Marshall, Jr., druggist.
- 1803 Malcolm McDonald, merchant.
- 1804 Sarah Moore.
- 1806 John Morton, Jr., merchant.
- 1807 Gouverneur Morris, of New York.
- " John Miller, butcher.
- 1810 John Mullowny.
- 1812 William Morrison, brewer.
- 1815 James Mease, M.D.
- 1816 John W. Moore, M.D.
- 1817 Samuel Mason, Steward Penn. Hospital.
- 1818 George Morris.
- " James J. Mazurie.
- 1819 Lloyd Mifflin.
- 1820 John Moore, M.D.
- 1821 William Montelius, tobacconist.
- " Elizabeth Marshall, druggist.
- 1825 J. K. Mitchell, M.D.
- 1826 Stephen P. Morris.
- " Charles D. Meigs, M.D.
- 1827 Caleb B. Mathews, M.D.
- 1831 John Moss, merchant.
- 1834 Caspar Morris, M.D.
- 1835 Thomas Mellon.
- 1836 Samuel George Morton, M.D.

1837 George McClellan, M.D.
1841 Isaac P. Morris, iron-founder.
" Jacob G. Morris.
1844 Wistar Morris, iron-founder.
" Henry Morris, iron-founder.
1845 Thomas H. McAllister, optician.
" William Y. McAllister, optician.
" Charles Moyer, druggist.
1846 Israel Morris.
1847 Conrad Meyer, piano manufacturer.
" John B. Myers.
1849 William G. Malin, Steward Penn. Hospital.
" Richard M. Marshall.
1852 Mary Marshall.
" George W. Morris.
1853 Samuel C. Morton.
1854 S. Weir Mitchell, M.D.
" James Markoe.
" Israel W. Morris.
" Catharine Morris.
1855 Samuel Mason.
1856 Morris, Tasker & Morris.
" Andrew Manderson.
" Benjamin Marshall.
" Dr. J. Wilson Moore.
" Dr. J. Forsyth Meigs.
" Isaac Meyer.
" McKean, Borie & Co.
" Catharine McCall.
" John Mason.
" Richards & Miller.
" Charles Megarge.
" Wm. L. Maddock.
" Charles Macalester.
" Richard C. McMurtrie.
" David Milne.
" James Martin.
" John McAllister, Jr.
" McAllister & Bro.
" James McGee.
" William R. Maxfield.
" Abram Miller.
" Mary Elizabeth Mackey.
1857 Samuel Morris.
" Morris, Jones & Co.
" William McCallum.
" Alex. R. McHenry.
" Joseph B. Myers.
" James Manderson.
" Thomas Manderson.
" Robert Morrell, M.D.
" A. Miskey.
" Charles McKeone.
" John S. Miller.
" Patrick McBride.
" Sons of Malta.
" Thomas H. Moore.
" Israel W. Morris, Jr.

1857 John M. Maris.
" Samuel V. Merrick.
" Thomas J. Magear.
" James McIlvain.
" Michael Molloy.
" Edward Maule.
" Israel Maule.
" Henry Maule.
" Charles McCandless.
" H. C. Megarge.
" A. J. McClure.
1858 Samuel Megargee.
" William Miller.
" C. H. Mattson.
" Robert V. Massey.
" Hugh McIlvain.
" William Musser.
" James A. McCrea, M.D.
" John R. Morrell.
" Dr. Samuel Moore.
" Megargee Bro.
" Hiram Miller.
1859 William H. Moore.
" John R. McCurdy.
" Malone & Taylor.
" Myers, Kirkpatrick & Co.
" Sarah Marshall.
" P. Pemberton Morris.
" William G Morehead.
" Harry McCall, Jr.
" James Mott.
" Anne D. Morrison.
" E. L. Moss.
" Joseph S Medara.
" Mahlon Moon.
" Jacob Miles & Son.
" Joel B. Morehead.
" David McConkey.
" John McAllister.
" Stephen Morris.
" Massey, Collins & Co.
1862 Dr. T. Geo. Morton.
1863 Merrick & Sons.
" Henry Pratt McKean.
1864 Thomas Mott.
" Morris, Wheeler & Co.
" McCallum & Co.
1865 Henry D. Moore.
" Samuel Mason, Jr.
" Thomas McEwen, M.D.
" John C. Mercer.
" George C. Morris.
" James T. Morris.
" Isaac W. Morris.
" John T. Morris.
" Lydia T. Morris.
" R. P. Morton.
1866 Levi Morris.
" Hannah Morris.
" Thomas Miller.

1867 James Moore & Son.
" Moore & Campion.
" E. P. Moyer & Bros.
" I. P. Morris, Towne & Co.
" Theo. Megargee & Co.
" Matthews & Moore.
" E. Spencer Miller.
" J. E. Mitchell.
" Helen K. Morton.
" J. H. Morris.
" James T. Magee.
" Michael H. Magee.
" William S. Magee.
" Thomas S. K. Morton.
" Mellor, Baines & Mellor.
" Miskey, Merrill & Thackara.
" Massey, Houstoun & Co,
" Jane Morris.
1868 J. Aitken Meigs, M.D.
1869 T. Magee & Co.
1874 Chas. M. Morton.
1876 Dr. Arthur V. Meigs.
" Edith Mason.
" Alfred C. Mason.

### N.

1751 Isaac Norris, Esq.
" Samuel Neave.
" Charles Norris.
" John Nelson.
" Samuel Noble.
1752 Peter Nygh.
1754 John Nixon.
1760 William Neate, of London.
1764 Richard Neave and Son, London.
1786 Alexander Nesbit.
" Philip Nicklin.
1794 Mary Norris.
1813 Joseph P. Norris.
1815 Henry Neill, M.D.
1818 George Nugent.
1822 Lindsay Nicholson.
1823 Joseph G. Nancrede, M.D.
1828 James S. Newbold.
1833 George W. Norris, M.D.
1845 Paul W. Newhall.
" John Notman
1856 Thos. A. Newhall.
" Charles Newbold.
" Newbold, Son & Aertson.
" Daniel Neall.
" Richard Norris.
" Thomas S. Newlin.
" Noblit, Brown & Noblit.
1857 Joseph A. Needles.
" James Nevins.
" Isaac Norris.
1859 Norcross & Sheets.

1859 James S. Newbold.
1860 Mrs. Robert Nelson.
1863 William F. Norris, M.D.
" J. Shipley Newlin.
" Thomas S. Newlin, Jr.
" Samuel Norris.
" Richard Norris & Son.
1865 Charles F. Norton.
1867 Newhall, Borie & Co.
" Richard L. Nicholson.
1871 Rev. Matthew Newkirk, Jr.
1873 N. P. S. (N. Parker Shortridge).

### O.

1751 John Ord, shopkeeper.
1758 Charles Osborne.
1759 Daniel Offley, smith.
1761 George Owen, hatter.
1762 John Oseland.
1766 Samuel Ormes, M.D.
1774 John Odenheimer, victualler.
1796 John Oldden.
1813 John C. Otto, M.D.
" Griffith Owen, clock and watchmaker.
1852 George Ord.
" Joseph B. Ord.
1856 J. B. Okie.
" Lewis G. Osbourne.
" Outerbridge, Harvey & Co.
" Charles S. Ogden.
" James H. Orne.
1857 John M. Ogden.
1858 Benjamin Orne.
" George R. Oat.
" Charles Oakford & Son.
1859 Margaret J. Otto.
1860 J. F. & E. B. Orne.

### P.

Thomas and Richard Penn (sons of Wm. Penn), an annuity of £10 paid from 1762 to 1775.
1751 Israel Pemberton, merchant.
" Israel Pemberton, Jr., merchant.
" Richard Peters, Esq.
" James Pemberton, merchant.
" William Plumstead.
" Edward Penington.
" John Pole.
1752 Samuel Powell, hatter.
" Thomas Paschall, hatter.
1754 John Pemberton.
" Oswald Peel.
" Joseph Parker.
" Richard Partridge, of London.

1754 William Parr, attorney-at-law.
1756 John Palmer, bricklayer.
" Isaac Paschall.
" John Parrish, bricklayer.
" Richard Pearne.
1757 William Peters, of Concord (in lumber).
1758 Samuel Purviance.
" Isaac Parrish.
" Joseph Paul, miller.
1759 Richard Parker.
" Samuel Powell.
1761 Thomas Penrose.
" James Penrose.
" John Paul, of Wissahickon, miller.
" William Pusey, merchant.
" John Potts, Esq.
1765 Charles Pettit.
1766 Nathaniel Pennock.
1767 Joseph Potts, merchant.
" Samuel Pleasants.
1768 Joseph Paschall.
" Samuel Potts.
1770 Joseph Pemberton.
1776 Thomas Parke, M.D.
1780 Jonathan Potts, M.D. (a loan office certificate for £1000).
1781 Frederick Phile, M.D.
1785 Timothy Pickering.
" John Pringle.
1786 Elliston Perot.
" Jeremiah Parker.
" Richard Parker.
" Michael Pragers.
" Ignatius Polyart.
1787 Derick Peterson.
" Thomas Penrose, Jr., shipbuilder.
" Henry Physick.
1788 John Penn.
" John Penn, Jr.
1790 John Perot, merchant.
1793 William Penrose.
1794 Philip S. Physick, M.D.
" Elizabeth Coates Paschall.
" Sarah Paschall.
1795 Zachariah Poulson, Jr.
" Thomas Paschall, merchant.
" Edward Penington, Jr., sugar-refiner.
" Isaac Penington, sugar-refiner.
" Israel Pleasants, merchant.
" Joseph Paschall, merchant.
1799 George Pennock, merchant.
1800 Abraham Patton, watchmaker.
1801 Henry Pratt.
" William Poyntell, merchant.
1804 Joseph Price, hatter.
1805 Samuel Parrish, merchant.
1807 Thomas Palmer, merchant.
1808 David Parrish.

1811 George Peterson.
1814 Henry Pemberton.
" Joseph M. Paul.
1815 Joseph Parrish, M.D.
1819 Isaac Parry, plasterer.
" William P. Paxson.
1821 William Price, M.D.
1822 Richard Price, Jr., merchant.
1825 John Paul.
1834 Abraham L. Pennock.
" Sansom Perot.
" Caspar W. Pennock.
1836 John Hare Powell (a calf).
1837 William Pepper, M.D.
1838 Edward Peace, M D.
1839 Joseph Pancoast, M D.
1840 Isaac Parrish, M.D.
1842 George Pepper, brewer.
1843 William Platt, merchant.
1845 Clayton T. Platt.
" Hannah Paul.
1846 Henry Pepper.
1848 Charles Collins Parker, M.D.
" Thomas H. Powers, chemist.
1852 Dr. Wm. Byrd Page.
" Eli K. Price.
" Joshua L. Price.
1853 Dillwyn Parrish.
1854 Caroline Pennock.
1855 Hannah Parke.
1856 Edward Perot.
" Charles Perot.
" John F. Peniston.
" Joseph Patterson.
" Francis Perot.
" Charles W. Pultney.
" William S. Perot.
" Joseph Perot.
" Robert Pearsall.
" Letitia Poultney.
" Sarah R. Paul.
1857 Palmer, Thomas & Co.
" Frederick S. Pepper.
" Henry M. Phillips.
" Prichett & Baugh.
" George D. Parrish.
" Elliston Perot.
" D. T. Pratt.
" Richard Price.
" Parry & Randolph.
" Edward T. Pusey.
" Samuel Parry.
" Ario Pardee.
" George Philler.
1858 Edward Patterson.
" Geo. W. Page.
" Francis Peters.
" Daniel R. Paul.
" Daniel R. Paul, Jr.
" Jonathan Palmer & Co.

1858 Wm. D. Parrish.
1859 Frances Pierpont.
" Robert S. Paschall.
" Thomas Potter.
" Thomas Pritchett.
" Asa Packer.
" A. Pardee & Co.
" David Potts, Jr.
" Stephen S. Price.
" Jane Preston.
" James W. Paul.
" A. M. Powers.
" Mrs. G. S. Pepper.
1860 Mrs. Morris Patterson.
" Mary Pepper.
" Sally W. Pennock.
" Mary T. Pleasants.
1861 John H. Packard, M.D.
" Wm. F. Potts.
1862 John H. Palethorpe, Est. of.
1864 J. Price Patton.
" R. Hare Powell.
" R. S. Peterson.
1865 William Pepper, Jr., M.D.
" Sarah Phipps.
" Caleb Peirce.
" Fannie R. Purves.
" William Platt Pepper.
" George S. Pepper.
" Philip Physic Peace.
" Edward Coleman Peace.
" Benjamin Perkins, Jr.
" Sarah A. Purves.
1867 Davis Pearson & Co.
" Moro Phillips.
" T. Morris Perot & Co.
" John Hare Powell.
" Mrs. John Hare Powell.
1868 William Procter, Jr.
1869 Est. of Davis Pearson, dec.
1870 William A. Porter.
" Mrs. S. N. Pepper.

Q.

1857 James W. Queen.

R.

1751 John Reynell.
" Hugh Roberts.
" Joseph Richardson, merchant.
" Francis Richardson.
" John Ross.
" John Redman, M.D.
" Samuel Rhoads.
1754 John Roberts, miller.
" Daniel Roberdeau.

1756 Peter Reeve
" Francis Rawle.
" Joseph Redman.
" Daniel Rundle.
" John Rhea
1757 Benjamin Rawle.
1758 John Relfe.
" William Rush, blacksmith.
" Isaac Roberts, brickmaker.
" John Rouse.
" John Rhobotham.
1759 Thomas Robinson, merchant.
1761 John Reily.
1763 Christopher Rawson, of Halifax.
" Nicholas Rittenhouse, miller.
1765 George Roberts.
" Samuel Rhoads, Jr.
" Thomas Ringold, of Maryland.
1766 Mary Richardson.
1767 Thomas Rutter.
" Thomas Robeson.
" Thomas Riché, merchant.
1768 Joseph Richardson, goldsmith.
1770 Benjamin Rush, M.D.
1786 Edward Russell.
" David Rittenhouse.
1787 Richard Rundle.
1788 James Read, flour merchant.
" George Rutter (picture of Good Samaritan).
1789 William Rawle.
1795 Robert Ralston, merchant.
1800 John Redman, M.D.
1801 John Robeson, merchant.
" William Redwood.
1802 Samuel Rhoads, merchant.
1806 Jacob Ridway, merchant.
1813 James Rush, M.D.
1814 William Rogers.
1815 Samuel Richards.
1821 Mark Richards.
1822 Hugh Roberts.
1823 Charles Roberts.
1828 William Rush, M.D.
" Jacob Randolph, M D.
1831 David Rankin, grocer.
1835 Romulus Riggs.
1841 Solomon W. Roberts, civil engineer.
" Elihu Roberts, merchant.
" Caleb C. Roberts, merchant.
1843 John J. Ridgway.
1845 Mrs. Hugh Roberts.
1849 Richard Ronaldson.
1851 Nathaniel Randolph.
1852 Mrs. M. Ricketts.
" Moncure Robinson.
" Jonathan Richards.
1855 Richard Ronaldson.
" Thomas Ridgeway.

1856 Hugh Roberts.
" Randolph & Jenks.
" John R. Rue.
" Thomas Robins.
" Charles P. Relf.
" Robert J Ross.
" Richard Richardson.
" Evans Rodgers.
" Thomas Richardson & Co.
" Edward Roberts.
" Evan Randolph.
" Richards & Miller.
1857 Charles W. Rogers.
" Philip S. Reilly.
" George W. Richards.
" Benjamin B. Reath.
" Samuel Rhoads.
" Rutter, Newhall & Co.
" Richardson, Thomas & Co.
" Anne R. Reynolds.
" John T. Ricketts.
" George D. Rosengarten.
" William B. Reed.
" Samuel Riddle.
" Wm. H. Richards.
" John G. Repplier.
1858 Clement S. Rutter.
" James Robb.
" Benjamin Rowland.
" John Robbins, Jr.
" A. S. & E. Roberts.
" William Rowland.
" John J. Richardson.
" Joseph J. Redner.
" John Rice.
" Joseph W. Ryerss.
1859 William L. Rehn.
" A. L. Randall.
" Richardson & Carver.
" Jacob Reigle.
" Charles Rugan.
" Mary Ashbridge Rhoads.
" Hannah Richardson.
" Charles Rhoads.
" Mrs. Thos. Robins.
1860 John Richardson.
" James Rowland & Co.
" Ritter & Brother
" Rockhill & Wilson.
" Elizabeth Rhoads.
1863 Samuel J. Reeves.
1864 R. N. Rathbun.
" William Rowland & Co.
" James Rowland.
" Nathan Rowland.
" Stephen Robbins.
" Dr. James E. Rhoads.
" John M. Read.
" Wm G. Rhoads.
" Edward Rhoads, M.D.

1865 Edward Taylor Randolph.
" Albert C. Roberts.
" John Robins.
" P. Reilley & Son.
" B. Howard Rand, M.D.
1866 Craig D. Richie.
1867 H. B. Rianhard.
" A. P. Roberts & Co.
" Wm. Reid.
" W. H. Rhaun.
" Lewis H. Redner.
" Wm. K. Ramborger.
" J. G & G. S. Repplier.
" Robert L. Reilly.
" Julianna Randolph.
1869 Joseph G. Richardson.
1872 Charles Roberts.
1874 John B. Roberts, M.D.


S.

1751 John Smith.
" Samuel Sansom.
" Edward Shippen.
" Thomas Stretch.
" Thomas Say.
1752 Christopher Sauer.
" Peter Sonmans, M.D.
" William Shipley, victualler.
" William Shippen, M.D.
1754 Stephen Shewell, baker.
" Joseph Shewell, baker.
" Jacob Shoemaker, Jr., wheelwright.
" Samuel Smith, merchant.
" William Smith, tanner.
" Robert Smith, carpenter.
" Isaac Snowden, tanner.
" William Stanley.
" Moses Stanley.
" Joseph Sennard.
" James Stone.
" James Stevenson.
" Daniel Steinmetz, baker.
" Samuel Swift.
" Valentine Stanley.
1755 Jacob Shoemaker, smith.
1756 Joseph Saunders.
" Joseph Stretch.
" Attwood Shute.
" Amos Strettell.
" John Stamper, Esq.
" Joseph Stamper.
1758 Edward Shippen, Jr
" William Shute, tallow-chandler.
" Thomas Saltar, lumber merchant.
" James Stoops, brickmaker.
" Enoch Story.
" Walter Shee, merchant.

1759 Barnaby Shute.
" John Scott, merchant.
1760 John Smith, of Kingsessing.
" Joseph Sermon, smith.
1761 John Shoemaker, of Cheltenham.
" Richard Smith, merchant.
" Joseph Sims.
" John Casper Stivers.
1762 Jedediah Snowden.
" Jonathan Shoemaker.
" George David Sickle, butcher.
1764 Adam Straker, smith.
1765 John George Snyder.
1766 William Shippen, Jr., M.D.
1767 Jonathan B Smith.
" Samuel Southall.
1768 William Sitgreaves, merchant.
" Samuel Sansom, Jr.
1771 Joseph Shippen, Jr.
" Joseph Stout.
" Robert Stevens.
" James Stewart, merchant.
1772 Joseph Swift.
1774 Samuel Simpson.
1775 Philip Syng.
1776 Jacob Spicer, of New Jersey.
1780 Benjamin Say, M.D.
1782 George Shoemaker, blacksmith.
1784 John Swanwick.
1785 Leonard Snowden.
" Lawrence Seckel, merchant.
" James Smith, Jr.
1786 Samuel Shaw.
" Robert Stevenson.
1787 Robert Smith, merchant.
" Townsend Speakman.
1794 Joseph Sansom.
" Thomas Stewardson.
1795 William Sansom, merchant.
1797 Jacob Shoemaker.
" Buckridge Sims.
1799 Charles Shoemaker.
" Esther Sprague, of Dedham, Mass.
1800 Willet Smith, merchant.
1801 Thomas Shoemaker, merchant.
" John Simpson, merchant.
" James Skerrett, blacksmith.
1802 Thomas Stewart.
" William W. Smith, merchant.
" James Stokes, merchant.
" James Smith, merchant.
1803 Stephen Smith, merchant.
" Philip Smith, grocer.
1806 George Smith, merchant.
1807 Thomas Shipley, merchant.
" James Stewart, M.D.
" John J. Smith, merchant.
" Daniel Sutter, grocer.
1811 John Savage, merchant.
1812 James Sawer.
1814 William Schlatter, merchant.
" Samuel Spackman, merchant.
" Ann Saunders, teacher.
1815 Joseph Allen Smith.
1816 John Stack.
" Charles J. Sutter.
1817 William A. Skerrett.
1818 Edward James Stiles.
1819 Nathan Shoemaker.
1820 Samuel Sellers.
1821 James Schott.
1830 John Struthers, marble-mason.
1833 Blakey Sharpless, bookseller.
1834 Samuel L. Shober.
" Benjamin P. Smith.
" John W. Shoemaker.
1835 Thomas Stewardson, M.D.
" Rebecca Simmons.
1837 George Roberts Smith.
1842 James Schott, Jr.
" George Stewardson.
" Rev. Edward J. Sourin.
1843 Alfred Stillé, M.D.
1844 Henry Seybert.
" Joseph Swift, broker.
1845 Alexander H. Smith.
" Isaac Starr.
1846 John Sergeant, attorney at-law.
1847 Henry H. Smith, M.D.
1848 C. E. Spangler.
" Robert W. Sykes.
" John Siter, merchant.
1849 Moreton Stillé, M D.
1851 Wm. Struthers, marble-mason.
" Joseph P. Smith.
1852 John P. Steiner.
" F. Sargeant, M.D.
" Henry G. Sharpless.
1855 Lewis A. Scott.
" Rosa Steadman.
" Dr. George Smith.
" Charles Sauter.
1856 Joseph Shipley.
" Catharine W. Sheppard.
" Samuel F. Smith.
" William S. Smith & Co.
" J. R. Savage & Co.
" Thomas M. Smith.
" John Saunders.
" Macpherson Saunders.
" John M. Scott.
" Jacob R. Smith.
" John M. Sharpless.
" Newberry A. Smith.
" Curwen Stoddart.
" Joseph M. Stoddart.
" Lindley Smyth.
" John Stone & Sons.
" Cornelius Stevenson.

1856 Daniel Smith, Jr.
" Robert H. Small.
" Frances W. Stevenson (N. Y.)
" Edward A. Smith, M.D.
" Joseph S. Silver.
" Wm. P. & A. Sharpless.
" James B. Shannon.
" Edwin Swift.
" Victor A. Sartori.
" Joseph J. Sharpless.
" Elwood Shannon.
" Edwin Spooner.
" William S. Spooner.
" Robert Shoemaker & Co.
1857 William L. Schaffer.
" Samuel E. Stokes.
" George H. Stewart.
" Thomas Sparks.
" Henry Sloan.
" Samuel R. Simmons.
" Stratton & Bro.
" John T. Smith.
" James S. Smith, Jr.
" William H. Stewart.
" James Schott.
" John S. Sharpless
" Stroup & Brother.
" Maria Stillé.
" Robert Steen.
" Enos Sharpless.
" William E. Stevenson.
" Samuel S. Scattergood.
" James Starr.
1858 Samuel Sloan.
" Gideon Scull.
" Isaac Starr, Jr.
" Stevens & Miller.
" Samuel Simes.
" Sharpless Bros.
" Alfred Slade & Co.
" Thos. Struthers.
" David Scull.
" Lawrence Shuster.
" Peter Sieger.
" Gottlieb Schiedt.
1859 Charles Shoemaker.
" J. & M. Saunders.
" Stewart & Patterson.
" Hannah Sansom.
" George B. Sloat.
" Richard G. Stotesbury.
" Dr. F. G. Smith.
" Stitt & Brown.
" John B. Shober.
" Samuel L. Shober.
" Joseph L. Schaffer.
" George R. Smith.
" William Sellers & Co.
" William Sellers.
" Jacob B. Shannon.

1859 David C. Spooner.
" Edward Sharpless.
" Edmund Smith.
" George K. Smith.
" Granville Stokes.
" Edward S. Simmonds.
" George P. Smith.
" Joseph Scattergood.
" Mrs. Nuberry Smith.
" Mrs. Geo. H. Stewart.
" John Stott.
" Abraham Scott.
" G. Washington Smith.
" Thomas A. Scott.
" Edmund Smith.
1860 Mrs. Isaac Starr.
" Misses Smith.
" Sellers & Pennock.
" Joseph W. Stokes.
" Townsend Sharpless.
" John J. Smith.
1864 Samuel R. Shipley.
" Wm. Savery, M.D.
" Sidney J. Sohns.
" Samuel J. Sharpless.
" Anna R. Sharpless.
" M. V. B. Sharpless.
" D. C. Wharton Smith.
" Adeline Margaret Sager.
" Thomas Smith.
" Isaac Sharpless.
" William B. Smith.
" Robert Pearsall Smith.
" Thomas Stillman.
1865 James D. Smith.
" E. A. Souder & Son.
" John F. Sheaff.
" William Stevenson.
" Charles Spencer.
" M. D. Shallcross, M.D.
" Alexander Simes.
" Isaac R. Smith.
" Abraham Schiedt.
1866 Albert H. Smith, M.D.
1867 Walter Smith.
" Rebecca Smith.
" Wm. F. Simes & Son.
" John Supplee.
" N. Parker Shortridge.
" Charles Smith.
" Curwen Stoddart, Jr.
" Robert Shoemaker.
" Benjamin H. Shoemaker.
" Smith, Randolph & Co.
" W. D. Smith & Co.
" William G. Spencer.
" Hon. William Strong.
1868 Thomas Shipley.
1869 William H. Sowers.
1870 Thomas Stewartson, Jr.

1870 Charles B. Shoemaker.
1871 Walter M. Spraukle.
1876 Henry J. Stout.
" Robert Shoemaker, Jr.
" Samuel B. Shoemaker.

### T.

1751 Robert Tuite.
1752 Joseph Trotter.
1754 Christopher Thompson.
" Peter Turner.
" Thomas Tillbury, baker.
1755 John Tinker, Governor of the Bahama Islands.
1756 John Taylor.
" Charles Thompson.
1761 Joseph Thomas, Flour Inspector.
" Joseph Turner, Esq.
1764 Robert Towers.
1765 John Test.
1767 James Tilghman.
1775 Alexander Todd.
1780 Dean Timmons.
1781 Robert Towers, M.D. (in medicines).
1785 Daniel Tyson.
1786 Peter Thompson, Jr., scrivener.
1787 Andrew Tybout.
1788 John Thompson, merchant.
1789 Richard Truman.
1795 Joseph Thomas, attorney-at-law.
1799 Henry Toland, grocer.
1801 Richard Tunis, merchant.
" Rev. James Taylor.
1802 Godfrey Twells, brewer.
1810 James Traquair.
1814 Jonah Thompson, merchant.
1815 James B. Thompson.
1817 George Thum.
" Edward Thompson, merchant.
" William Thackara.
" James Allen Thackara.
1819 A. B. Tucker, M.D.
1820 Benjamin Tucker, teacher.
1844 Thomas T. Tasker, iron-founder.
" William P. Tatham.
1845 George Thomas.
" Jacob M. Thomas.
1847 John Towne.
1852 Thomas T. Tasker, Jr.
" Joseph R. Tasker.
" George Thomas, M.D.
" John R. Thomas.
1856 Edward H. Trotter.
" William Henry Trotter.
" Charles W. Trotter.
" Job R. Tyson.
" John Trucks.

1856 Est. of Jno. R. & Geo. Thomas.
" Jane Thomas.
" John D. Taylor.
" Tatham Brothers.
" John J. Thompson.
" Joseph W. Taylor, M.D.
" Joseph C. Turnpenny.
" Charles Taylor.
" John H. Towne.
" John R. T. & George Thomas.
" Thain & McKeon.
" George Townsend.
" Frederick A. Tupper.
1857 George E. Taylor.
" Benjamin T. Tredick.
" Newcomb B. Thompson.
" William Taylor.
" Thurlow Hughes & Co.
" David Thaine.
1858 George H. Thompson.
" Henry Tilge & Co.
" William and Geo. Thompson.
" Taylor, Gillespie & Co.
" Virginia Taylor (Norfolk).
" J. Edgar Thompson.
" Moses Thomas.
" Moses Thomas & Son.
" Joseph B. Townsend.
1859 George W. Taylor.
" Michael Trump & Son.
" Geo. Thompson.
" Paul Thurlo.
" Mary A. Taylor.
" Henry C. Townsend.
" Dr. Isaac Thomas.
" Nathan Taylor.
" Wm G. Thomas.
" Tessiere, Mrs.
" Mrs. B. Taylor.
1860 Solomon Townsend.
" Joseph M. Thomas.
1861 Thomas Thompson.
1864 Lewis Thompson & Co.
" George Trotter.
" Edward Tatum.
1865 Chas. P. Tutt, M D.
" Richard S. Thomas.
" William P. Tatham.
" Susan T. Thompson.
" James B. Thompson.
" Charles T. Thompson.
" John J. Thompson, Jr.
" George F. Taylor.
1866 John Thompson, Jr.
" Lewis Taws.
1867 Joseph Trimble.
" Lydia Thomas.
" E. G. Townsend.
" Geo. M. Troutman.
" Henry B. Tatham.

1867 Geo. N. Tatham.
" Henry Tilge.
" George Trott.
1869 George Tales.
1873 Elizabeth R. Turnpenny.
" Rebecca A. Tasker.
1876 Mary E. Turnpenny.

## U.

1769 Abraham Usher.
1856 George Urwiler.

## V.

1756 William Vanderspiegel.
1761 John Vanderen.
1785 John Vaughan.
1786 William Von Phul.
1796 Ambrose Vasse, merchant.
1799 William Vicary, mariner.
1819 Roberts Vaux.
1826 George Vaux.
1837 F. A. Vandyke, M.D.
1855 Eliza H. Vaux.
" W. S. Vaux.
1856 George Vaux, Jr.
" Mrs. S. B. Vansycle.
" Verree & Mitchell.
1859 Vandevear & Bolton.
" Charles Vezin.
1867 Wm. P. Vaux.

## W.

1751 Casper Wistar.
" Joseph Wharton, cooper.
" Townsend White, merchant.
" Robert Willan.
1752 John Wistar.
" James Wright.
" Daniel Williams, baker.
1754 Charles West.
" John Wier.
" Abraham Wagner.
" Robert Waln, merchant.
" Richard Wistar.
" Joseph Watkins.
" George Westcott, brazier.
" Charles West, Jr., cooper.
" Anthony Wilkinson, carver.
" Joseph Wills, clockmaker.
" Edmund Winder.
" Jacob Winey.
" Joseph Wood, merchant.
" Peter Worrell.

1755 Jeremiah Warder, hatter.
1756 William Wallace.
" Thomas Wharton.
" James Whitehead.
" James Wharton.
" Joseph Wharton, Jr.
" Stephen Wooley.
" Samuel Wharton.
1758 William West, merchant.
" Stephen Williams.
" Swen Warner.
" James Wallace.
" William Wishart.
1759 Daniel Wistar.
" Joseph Warner.
1761 James West.
" Richard Waln.
" John Wood, clockmaker.
" Thomas Willing, Esq.
1762 John Whitelock.
" Isaac Whitelock.
" John Wikoff.
" James Webb.
" John Wilcocks.
" Joseph Watkins, Jr.
1763 Joseph Wetherill.
" Rev. George Whitfield.
1765 Thomas Wharton.
" Thomas Wagstaff, of London (a watch).
" James White.
1767 Richard Walker.
1768 Robert Wickersham.
1769 Joseph Watson, M.D.
" William Wistar.
1771 Anna Warner.
" Thomas Wishart, chandler.
" John Wharton.
1772 Benjamin Wynkoop.
" Jeremiah Warder, Jr.
1775 Richard Willing.
" Isaac Wharton.
" William Whitpain, carpenter.
1776 Noah Webster (lectures for benefit of hospital).
1780 Charles Wharton, merchant.
1782 John Wall.
1784 Samuel Williams, cabinet-maker.
1785 Christian Wirtz.
" William Wirtz.
" William West.
" Thomas Wistar.
" Israel Wheelen.
" Nicholas Waln.
1786 Gideon Hill Wells.
" Jesse Waln.
" John Warner, whalebone-carver.
" Henry Wynkoop.
" Solomon White.
" Robert Wharton.

1786 Philip Wager and George Habacker.
" Lambert Wilmer.
" James Wilson, shopkeeper.
" Charles West, Jr.
" Robert Waln, Jr., merchant.
" Sarah Wistar.
1787 Samuel Wheeler.
" Bartholomew Wistar.
1788 Richard Wistar.
" John Warder.
1791 Bryan Wilkinson.
" Caspar Wistar, M.D.
1795 Kearney Wharton, merchant.
" Caspar Wistar, of Chester Co.
" Catherine Wistar, Jr.
" George G. Woelpper, butcher.
1796 James Woodhouse, M.D.
1797 Dr. John White, druggist.
1798 Andrew Wood.
1799 Martha Whitelock.
1801 William Wister, merchant.
" William Waln, merchant.
1802 James Wood, merchant.
1803 Jeremiah Warder, Jr., merchant.
1806 John G. Wachsmuth, merchant.
" Alexander Wilson, merchant.
" Thomas M. Willing, merchant.
" John Watson.
1807 William Warner, merchant.
" Benjamin C. Wilcocks, merchant.
1808 Samuel Williamson, silversmith.
1810 George S. Wilson.
" John Wister.
" Charles J. Wister.
1811 Henry L. Waddell.
1812 Joseph Watson, lumber merchant.
1814 Israel Whelen.
1816 Jacob S. Waln, Jr.
" Edward Wilson.
1817 Benjamin West (picture of Christ Healing the Sick).
1819 Richard Wistar, Jr.
1821 Thomas Wildon.
" Silas E. Weir.
" Bartholomew Wistar.
1824 Caspar Wistar, M.D.
" Charles Watson.
1825 George B. Wood, M.D.
1828 Henry J. Williams, attorney-at-law.
1832 David Woelpper, Sr., butcher.
" Jeremiah Willets, plasterer.
1833 Josiah White.
1834 Captain William West, mariner.
" Henry White.
1835 Mifflin Wistar, M D.
" Joseph Warrington, M.D.
1840 Joshua M. Wallace, M.D.

1840 John Wistar, lumber merchant.
" B. Wyatt Wistar, merchant.
1841 Richard Willing.
1844 Charles Willing, M.D.
1845 Horatio C. Wood, merchant.
" John R. Worrell.
" William Welsh.
1846 Samuel Welsh.
" David Woelpper, Jr , butcher.
" George Woelpper, butcher.
1848 Robert F. Walsh.
" William Weightman, manufacturing chemist.
" Thomas H. White.
1851 Richard D. Wood, merchant.
" John M. Whitall.
1852 James Whitall.
1853 Charles S. Wurtz.
1854 R. Sterling Wilson.
" Edward S. Whelan.
" Peter Williamson.
" Henry J. Williams.
1855 S. Morris Waln.
" Rebecca White
1856 J. Ringgold Wilmer.
" Benjamin H. Warder.
" Elizabeth Wistar.
" Isaac S. Waterman.
" Dilwynn Wistar.
" Caleb Cresson Wistar.
" Bartholomew Wistar.
" G. D. Wetherill & Co.
" C. R. & S. Welsh.
" Charlotte W. Wetherill.
" Rachel P. Wetherill.
" Thomas B Wattson.
" John W. Wallace.
" Francis R. Wharton.
" Edward S. Whelan.
" Welsford & Wilson.
" Mrs. Samuel Welsh.
" Benjamin P. Williams.
" Samuel Williams.
" Thomas R. Williams.
" Isabella Williams.
" Asa Whitney & Sons.
" Wm. Woodnut.
" John R. Wilmer.
" Joseph Warner.
" Isaac S. Williams.
" Albert Worrell.
" John C. Weber.
" Tobias Wagner.
" Bathmel Wilson.
" Samuel Walley.
" Geo. W. Watson.
1857 Ambrose White.
" William Warner, Jr.
" George M. Warner.
" Harriet Warner.

1857 Catharine A. Warner.
" Thomas F. Wharton.
" Mahlon Williamson.
" William S. Wilson.
" David S. Winebrenner.
" George J. Weaver.
" Waterman, Osborne & Co.
" William R. White.
" John Wise.
" Charles Wise.
" John Wright.
" James D. Wetham.
" John Woodside & Co.
" Thomas Williamson.
" Isaiah V. Williamson.
" R. A. and J. J. Williams & Co.
" Howard Williams.
" James M. Wilcox & Co.
" John Welsh.
1858 John Wiegand.
" Mary Ann Williams.
" E. S. Whelan & Co.
" Wm Wilson & Sons.
" William Wainwright.
" Robert Whitaker.
" Morris S. Wickersham.
" Ellerslie Wallace.
" C. W. Warnick.
" D. N. Wetzler.
" Weaver & Volkner.
1859 J. V. Watson.
" Robert West.
" David Woelpper.
" Mary Wagner.
" John Werst.
" J. T. Way.
" Passmore Williamson.
" O. Howard Wilson.
" George F. Womrath.
" Warner, Miskey & Merrill.
" William Wilstach.
" James A. Wright.
" Richard Wright.
" George A. Wright.
" Samuel Wright.
" Jos. P. Wilson, of West Chester.
" John R. Walker.
" Wetherill & Bro.
" John Welsh, Jr.
" Mrs. Asa Whitney.
" Geo. D. Wetherill.
" John R. Worrell.
" Mark Wilcox.
" Wise, Pusey & Wise.
" Thomas Wilson, M.D.
" Mary R. Welsh.
" Anna M. Welsh.
" Mary Whitall.
" C. B. Wright.
" R. J. Watson.

1859 Mrs. Charles Wood.
" Samuel Watt.
1860 George Wrinler.
" Sarah Wistar.
" Workmen Factory of Code, Hopper & Gratz.
" James P. Wilson.
" Henry R. Worthington, of N. Y.
" Rebecca M. Welsh.
" Josephine E. Welsh.
" Wood & Perot.
1863 Lewis T. Wattson.
1864 Dr. Ellwood Wilson.
" Work, McCouch & Co.
" Richard D. Wood & Co.
" Joseph Wharton.
" Gideon G. Wescott.
" Charles W. Wharton.
" Edward M. Wright.
" Whitall, Tatum & Co.
" Henry L. Waln.
" Edward Waln.
1865 Annie Waln.
" Henry Wharton.
" Horace Williams.
" John R. Wercherer.
" Thomas Wistar, M.D.
" Geo. B. Wood.
" Horatio C. Wood, Jr., M D.
" John B. Wood.
" James F. Wood.
" William E. Wood.
" Caleb Wood.
1866 Alex. Whillden & Sons.
1867 Whelan, Townsend & Co.
" John R. White & Son.
" Henry Wallace.
" Sallie N. Waln.
" John H. Williams.
" Charles Wheeler.
" R. & G. A. Wright.
" Samuel J. White.
1868 Joseph Lapsley Wilson.
" Richard Wood.
1870 Redwood F. Warner.
" Charles H. Wagner.
1872 S. D. Walton.
" Wm. Wynne Wistar.
1873 George Watson.
1875 Jane G. Wilson.

Y.

1754 Francis Yarnall.
1756 Thomas York.
1776 William Young, potter (in earthernware).
1781 Peter Yarnall, M.D.
1785 Ellis Yarnall, merchant.

| | |
|---|---|
| 1807 Samuel Yorke. | 1860 Yarnall & Cooper. |
| 1813 Benjamin H. Yarnall, iron-monger. | 1867 James T. Young. |
| 1856 Charles Young. | |
| " Alexander Young. | Z. |
| " Charles Yarnall. | |
| 1857 William H. Yeaton. | 1754 Lloyd Zachary. |
| " William J Young. | " Isaac Zane. |
| " Mary Ann Yardley. | " Jonathan Zane. |
| 1858 Edward Yarnall. | 1759 Nathan Zane. |
| 1859 Yard, Gilmore & Co. | 1777 Isaac Zane, Jr. |
| " Howard Yarnall. | 1792 William Zane. |

## THE CONTRIBUTIONS OF THE PENN FAMILY.

Thomas and Richard Penn, sons of the distinguished founder of Pennsylvania, contributed (1762 to 1775) nearly $1500 to the purposes of this charity ; and, further, by patent dated November 10, 1767, gave, to complete the Hospital square, a lot of ground, extending on Spruce Street, from 8th to 9th Streets, 396 feet, and southwards a depth of 107 feet on 8th and 9th Streets respectively. They likewise gave to the Hospital, by patent dated in 1769, a lot on Spruce Street, extending west from 9th Street, 198 feet, and southwardly in depth 107 feet to other land of the Hospital; being part of the lot on which Portico Square is now built.

Contributions to this charity are received by John T. Lewis, Treasurer, or either of the Managers or Stewards.

Bequests should be made in the corporate name, to "THE CONTRIBUTORS TO THE PENNSYLVANIA HOSPITAL."

www.ingramcontent.com/pod-product-compliance
Lightning Source LLC
Chambersburg PA
CBHW030342170426
43202CB00010B/1213